Single and Satisfied

Single and Satsified

A grace-filled calling for the unmarried woman

Nancy Wilson

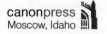

canonpress
Moscow, Idaho

To Bessie
who taught me that contentment is
a deep satisfaction with the will of God.

Elizabeth Catherine Dodds Wilson, 1919–2010

This second edition to my ten beautiful granddaughters:
*Jemima, Belphoebe, Hero, Lucia, Ameera, Lina, Daphne, Chloe,
Marisol, and Blaire.*

Published by Canon Press
P.O. Box 8729, Moscow, ID 83843
800-488-2034 | www.canonpress.com

Nancy Wilson, *Single and Satisfied: A grace-filled calling for the unmarried woman*
Copyright © 2021 by Nancy Wilson.
First published in 2010 under a different title.

Cover design by Rachel Hoffmann.
Printed in the United States of America.

Library of Congress Cataloging-in-Publication Data
Wilson, Nancy, 1952- author.
Single and satisfied : a grace-filled calling for the unmarried
    woman / Nancy Wilson.
Why isn't a pretty girl like you married?
Second edition. | Moscow, Idaho : Canon Press, [2021]
LCCN 2021017241 | ISBN 9781952410970 (paperback)
LCSH: Single women—Life skills guides. | Single women—United
    States—Life skills guides. | Single women—Religious life.
Classification: LCC HQ800.2 .W55 2021 | DDC 646.70082—dc23
LC record available at https://lccn.loc.gov/2021017241

21 20 19 18 17 16 15 14 13   9 8 7 6 5 4 3 2

Contents

Introduction... 9

CHAPTER 1
Taking Offense 13

CHAPTER 2
Is This an Affliction?............................19
And if it is, what do I do about it?

CHAPTER 3
Unmarried Women in the Covenant Community 23

CHAPTER 4
What about Dad? 31

CHAPTER 5
Is This Really God's Best?........................37

CHAPTER 6
Don't Be a Basket Case............................43

CHAPTER 7
Don't Pretend to Be Happy........................47

CHAPTER 8
Cheerfulness is Good Medicine 57

CHAPTER 9
Dressing with a Worldview........................63

CHAPTER 10
What Kind of Man Are You Looking For?............69

CHAPTER 11
Keep Your Heart................................75

CHAPTER 12
Are You Desirable? 81

CHAPTER 13
Loving the Brothers 87

CHAPTER 14
Loving the Competition 91

CHAPTER 15
Setting Standards of Personal Holiness 95

CHAPTER 16
Culture Building and the Single Woman............101

CHAPTER 17
Beauty in Your Home 107

CHAPTER 18
What About a Career?...........................113

CHAPTER 19
No Regrets 117

Introduction

Years ago my husband and I were attending a church dinner where part of the program included asking all the singles in the church to stand. At that time there were only three, my oldest daughter and two young men. When my daughter's turn came to be introduced, my husband said, "She's not single. She's a daughter!"

Ever since that evening, I have felt uncomfortable with the term *single* when referring to unmarried men and women in our church. Today our numbers have swollen, and we have many unmarried men and women of "marriageable age" as part of our growing church community. Our individualistic culture wants to label unmarried people as *singles,* but in the covenant community of God, there are no *singles.* God calls us family: brothers and sisters, mothers and fathers in Christ. We are each to be wonderfully connected to the other as part of a church community, where each person is needed and attached to others in her own family as well as to the broader church family.

In a healthy church community there will, of course, be many married couples with children of various ages; but there will also be widows, couples who do not have children, old people, college students, and unmarried men and women. In our church it is not uncommon for us to attend several baby or wedding showers a month. It's very easy to focus on the needs of these young women who are becoming wives or mothers, and forget to look out for the needs of the widows, childless couples, elderly saints, or the single men and women. This is why we need to stir one another up to love and good deeds. We are to minister to one another in various ways, and if we were all the same, life would be boring indeed. Fruit is never uniform; it is scattered about, some branches more heavily laden than others. Fruit is messy, but it is delightful. The church community is much the same. A single woman is just as much a part of the covenant community as the mother with ten children. And she can be just as fruitful as the mother with the large family, even if her fruit doesn't look the same. In the providence of God, each of us has a unique place among the saints.

Still, even if we adopt the common terminology and call unmarried women *singles*, we have to stop treating them as singles. My point here is to remember they are part of the covenant community and not unconnected to the rest of us. This requires wisdom for all the church, because the women in this category have a difficult time today finding their place in the world as well as in the church community. They can feel a very real pressure and expectation to get married. Many of the saints make well-meaning (but thoughtless) comments that exert this sort of pressure.

Another difficulty is the emphasis in the church on *family*. This is as it should be, for God designed the family as one of His great blessings to us. However, when so much of the church's good, biblical teaching revolves around being a godly wife and mother, an unmarried woman can wonder what she is supposed to be doing with her life. What is her role in the church? Does she have a purpose if she is unmarried? Is it just to look for a husband? Should she pursue a career? Unless the single women are instructed carefully and encouraged regularly, they can fall prey to discontent, self-pity, or anxiety, and they can fade into the woodwork, feeling a little useless.

To make single people feel like a part of the church, some churches start ministries to singles or have career groups that meet regularly for fellowship. Of course, this is not necessarily a bad thing itself, unless the group is devoted to silly skits and junior-high level games. But even if it is a sound group, it can become unhealthy if the only regular contact the unmarried women have with the church family is with their own peer group of "singles." These women need to be integrated into the families within the church. We are designed to fellowship with all age groups, babies to grannies, and we should not become exclusively attached to our "group." A Christian culture integrates everyone, young and old, married and unmarried, into the life of the church.

God did not design His people to live as "singles." We are to live as families even if we are not under the same roof. An unmarried woman should have a high view of marriage, but she should also have a high view of God's sovereignty in her own life. He directs our steps, He establishes our ways, and He certainly decrees when and if and to whom each woman is to be married. He does all things well. Whether a woman is called to singleness for a short time or for her whole life, she is called to be fruitful in God's kingdom. She is called to glorify and enjoy God with her whole heart. She is called to grow in grace and faith and to be of great use to the kingdom of God. Marriage is a means, not an end. It is one of the means God uses to glorify His name among us, but it is not His only means.

All of Scripture is given to all of us. The passages in the Bible that speak to women, speak to married and unmarried alike, though points of application may differ. The unmarried woman is to rejoice in her calling before the Lord. She is to be virtuous. She must cultivate a biblical femininity, be modest and pure, and overcome the hindrances to fulfilling her feminine calling. She must love the sisters and view marriage as a good thing. And best of all, she is to walk before her Lord in humility and hope, growing in faith and love as a vital part of the covenant community.

If the Christian community quits thinking of and treating the unmarried women simply as *singles,* that would be a great start. But you unmarried women yourselves have to do the same thing. You have to get a new mindset about this. It certainly requires that we all have wisdom. The single woman can be confused about her place in the world, in her family, and in her church community. I assume that most single women want to be married. Those who have the gift of celibacy don't want to be married, so they would not be the ones to pick up a book like this one. So I want to discuss some issues that need to be addressed, even if no one is else is talking about them. My desire in writing this book is to help the unmarried women in the church feel secure about who they are in Christ, and walk in His grace. And I also hope that the rest of us will grow in our understanding, so we can support, strengthen, encourage, and enjoy these unmarried saints.

CHAPTER 1

Taking Offense

No doubt we have all heard people say rude things to single women. Even worse, maybe we have said rude things ourselves. Single women, depending on how long they have been in the "still not married" category, could no doubt make an impressive list of thoughtless comments spoken to them by well-meaning people, often at social gatherings, and especially at friends' weddings. The old standby is, "Why isn't a pretty girl like you married?" It's a compliment, right? But it's also a nosey question. The women who have been the recipients of such comments should try to attribute the best of motives. Most of the time people are trying to be funny, or they are trying to make conversation, and it is all they can think of to say. We really must think the best of them. Taking offense at insensitive comments only makes for bitter women. If you can quickly bring to mind a list of people who have said unkind things about your unmarried state, perhaps you need to confess some hard feelings and bitterness. Let it go.

If we are going to talk about single women living in community with lots of married people, we have to be determined from the outset that we must all get along. And we must even do better than that: we must love one another and be quick to forgive. I suggest that you accept the fact that people, even dear, sweet, Christian people, can say and do atrocious things. And if they weren't saying stupid things that hurt your feelings about being single, then they would be saying something else that would be a temptation. Married women are not immune to such things. So realize that this is just a fact of life, and until the world changes, we will all be exposed to comments that are either deliberately rude at worst, or at best thoughtless and unkind. We might as well determine now that we will handle this like Christian women. And how exactly is that?

First of all, handle it with grace. A gracious spirit answers with gracious words. Peter tells us that "the Lord is gracious" (1 Pet. 2:3); Christ was known as gracious (Lk. 4:22), and Ecclesiastes says that "The words of a wise man's mouth are gracious, but the lips of a fool shall swallow him up" (10:12). It is easy to be annoyed or offended. We don't need grace to do that. But it requires grace from God to return good for evil, to overlook an insult, and to respond to an unkind comment with kindness. We are God's people; we must imitate Him in this.

Sometimes we really are too hard on others. They meant no harm. They did not realize it would hurt your feelings. They thought they were being friendly or funny. In fact, they meant it as a compliment! After all, they said you were pretty. But our tendency is to take it hard. We immediately attribute motives and assume they were intending to hurt us. This is where we have to lighten up a little and have a sense of humor about it. People generally are insensitive and say stupid things without thinking. That is why the Scriptures are so full of exhortations about the tongue. Assume that for each hurtful comment you have ever received, you have probably spoken at least a dozen to others. This will then give you a spirit of humility yourself. Let others' unkind comments be sermons to you, teaching you to be far more sensitive and caring to others than you have been before.

When saying this, I am not pretending that comments like these are no big deal. I know they are hurtful, unkind, insensitive, rude, and unloving. They can cause discouragement, embarrassment, annoyance, and even bring on tears. They can easily stumble you and lead to self-pity or cause you to doubt the Lord's mercy toward you. My point is not that these comments are no big deal. Rather, I want to encourage you to learn to deal with them with grace and wisdom. You want to process them like a Christian woman, not like a worldly woman. Sometimes half the battle is recognizing what is happening. If you can see it coming and identify it as a temptation, then you can ask God to give you a gracious answer and not stew about it later, thinking about all the very witty things you could have said to put that person in his place! If you know this is a stumbling block, and it is, then pray preventively that God will keep you from temptation. Then you can go with a sense of humor, wondering who it will be this time to make the witty crack.

This is a universal problem. Cancer patients hear horror stories from well-meaning friends about so-and-so who died a quick death after being diagnosed with the same disease. Pregnant women hear about terrible deliveries. When I was pregnant with my first baby, a well-meaning friend asked me who my doctor was. When I told her, she replied, "He almost killed my cousin!" And then she went on to tell the gory details. If you are building a house, you will hear horror stories about other people building houses. So naturally, if you are single, people will give you unhelpful, single comments. Why do we do this to one another? I surely do not know. It must be our first instinct, but we should know better. But we recognize it far better when others do it to us than when we are doing it to others. So cultivate humility in this area and pray for a gracious tongue. And don't assume that you are the only person who has to deal with this. We have received grace, so we extend it to others.

A gracious spirit also requires a lively sense of humor. Don't take it all so very seriously, even though the questions may be awkward. So many single women are asked very sticky questions, often from people they don't even know very well. First of all, you don't have to answer them. Just because a person asks you a very personal question does not mean you are required to give an answer. And of course it is better not to answer at all than to tell an outright lie. "Do you wish you were married?" someone might ask. Now, don't lie about it and say, "Oh, not really. I'm very happy with my life." What you really might want to say is, "What a stupid question!" But perhaps a gracious answer would be something like, "Do I ever!" And if you feel chatty, you can go on to say something like, "But I want to be married to the *right man*. I don't want to be married just to be married."

On the other hand, someone may ask a question that is way too personal. "Is anyone pursuing you right now?" "Is there anyone you are interested in?" "Have you ever been proposed to?" It may even be more specific and sticky. "What do you think of Brian? He's an eligible bachelor." Of course you may answer these if you want to. But an answer is not required. Why not laugh and say, "Do you really think I would answer such a question? No way!" Answering or not answering is perfectly acceptable. The one thing that is not acceptable is taking offense. Change the subject! You decide if it is someone you want to confide in or not.

Sometimes the well-meaning ladies in church will tell you they are praying for you. Say, "Thank you for thinking of me!" Be grateful for their kindness and don't let it ruffle you. After all, if you do want to be married, isn't it great to know people are praying for you in this? In our congregation, a few of the older Christian women have dedicated themselves to praying for spouses for all the singles, both men and women. They are serious about this, and they rejoice when they can "scratch a name off the list." This is not insensitive or crass. It is real Christian love.

Sometimes friends will want to press you to meet someone or ask you what you think of someone. The same principle applies here. Answer the questions that you are comfortable with. But don't allow prying questions to force you to make your private feelings public. And welcome help that really is help. There is no sin in trying to get unmarried people to meet each other, and no sin in wanting to meet each other. Don't over-spiritualize this process. My parents met on a blind date, and they are not unusual in this. Take all the help offered, if it is really going to be help. But feel free to pass when you know it won't really be the kind of help you want.

Finally, don't let comments like, "Why isn't a pretty girl like you married?" keep you from attending weddings or other social gatherings. You need to participate in community life. You need all these people (even if they are insensitive), and they need you. Realize that each comment has come with God's permission and view it as part of your sanctification. Learn to be more gracious in your own conversation so that you are not asking nosey questions yourself. And if the Lord permits you the opportunity, graciously tell them that such questions really make you uncomfortable.

CHAPTER 2

Is This an Affliction?

And if it is, what do I do about it?

One of the things I want to address in this book is the need to come face to face with reality and quit pretending that being unmarried is lots of fun. In some cases, it may be. And in other cases, it is a phony show. On one hand, single women are encouraged to be content in their circumstances and to trust that this is "God's best" for them; on the other hand, they are urged to view their unmarried state as an affliction from which they are seeking deliverance. So which is right?

I believe that being single can certainly be an affliction for those who are not gifted with celibacy. It was not a hardship for the apostle Paul. But for someone without that calling, it is a hardship and may be a form of suffering, depending on the circumstances. If being unmarried really is an affliction for you, then Scripture has much to say about how you are to view it, and we'll consider some of those things shortly. If a woman who longs for marriage and does not have the gift of celibacy pretends that her life is easy, she will not find the help from God's Word that is available to her.

At the same time, some women really do not feel *afflicted*. They are busy, fruitful, and truly contented, though they do pray for a husband. All women are different, and they handle things differently, so I am hesitant to call the unmarried state an affliction across the board. For some, it truly is.

When I was single and out of college, I had a friend who viewed her singleness as an affliction indeed. She spoke of it constantly, and I remember her working on some needlework and saying, "When I get married, I'm going to tell my husband, *'I did this while I was waiting for you!'*" Everything she did was in relation to waiting for her husband. I remember disliking her viewpoint and wanting to adopt a different one. I remember thinking it over and determining that I wanted to have a different perspective. I didn't want to be "waiting around." I wanted to be *going* somewhere. I did not want to view my time as simply treading water, always waiting for something to happen. I thought that I should be moving forward in my Christian life, believing that God would bring someone into my life along the way.

Now I think both perspectives are lawful. I think I was happier than my friend, but I don't think she was necessarily in sin because she was constantly thinking about marriage. But she wasn't always fun to be around. She got married a few years later, and I wonder if she had the same attitude about having children. And then about the next thing and the next. We establish patterns that are hard to break.

I assumed that I would eventually be married, and I prayed regularly, not for *a* husband, but for *my* husband, whoever he was. I knew that God knew who he was, even if I didn't. So I prayed that he would be growing in faith and walking with God. I had lonely times like everyone else. I had temptations to get impatient.

At the same time, I wanted to have direction and purpose, and I wanted that purpose to be maturing in the faith, growing in my Christian life. So I tried to attend as many Bible studies and conferences as I could, knowing that after I was married that would not be as easy to do. I remember telling myself that I did not want to look back with regret, wishing I had trusted God more, wishing that I had been more at peace.

This is where we have to allow for different personalities. Some are more naturally optimistic than others. This is not to be confused with godliness! For some single women, it is a heavy burden to be waiting to be married. For others it may not be as difficult. But we need to look at our own temptations and determine to have a plan to overcome them. In Christ we can do this.

If being unmarried is an affliction, then the Christian woman can see it as part of God's sanctifying work in her life. She can know that God is teaching her, that she is enrolled in a class, and that she wants to get good grades so she can pass on to the next level. All women have temptations. If we are unmarried, we have unmarried temptations; if we are married, we have married temptations. No one is free from temptation. So we look for our duties as laid out in God's Word to us, and we do the next thing. We are to pray for deliverance, and we are to trust the Lord and rejoice in Him.

Some women feel guilty about praying for a husband. They wonder if they should just give up and at what age they should "accept" their singleness, period. The person in an affliction should persevere in prayer, all the while trusting that God is using the affliction for good. It is foolish to quit praying, unless the prayer itself is a snare to your soul, causing you to be more miserable and worrisome about your situation. That is a sign that the praying isn't really productive, and must not be the prayer of faith.

But the woman who can pray for her future husband with a spirit of expectancy and longing, all of which is joyfully submitted to God, should never give up praying. The only time to quit asking for a husband is when you cease to want one.

A single woman should not sit around like a bump on a log waiting for a godly husband to fall out of the sky. In the following chapters, I will discuss some of the things a woman can do to improve her attitude, her looks, her personality, and her spiritual life. These are all lawful things to make a woman happier and more content, as well as making her more desirable to a godly man. But she also has to get out of her house and meet people. I have heard single women complain about the fact that the single men never include them in their get-togethers. But when I asked these same women about the parties given by the same men that were general invitations to the whole church, they confessed that they hadn't gone. This is like going to the doctor, refusing to take the prescription, and then complaining that going to the doctor was a waste of time.

If being unmarried is an affliction for you, then look to the Bible and see all it has to say about affliction. There are many promises for you. Lay hold of them. Don't compare your afflictions to the afflictions of others. Learn to carry your own load, and give that load to Jesus. God has given you sweet consolation in Christ.

CHAPTER 3

Unmarried Women in the Covenant Community

It's tempting to think that there really isn't a niche for the single women in the church. The married women have their hands full with helping their husbands. The mothers have a big job managing their homes and rearing their children. Scripture lays out the duties of wives and mothers clearly, and the church provides plenty of teaching and instruction on the family. Sermons on marriage, books on courtship and childrearing, conferences for wives and husbands seem to occupy a central place in the work of the church. And of course, these are very important issues and need to be addressed. But the single woman can feel at sea in all this. If she is not engaged, what is she doing really? Does everyone assume she is biding her time waiting to get married? Is that necessarily bad? What is she supposed to be doing?

Actually, many Scriptures address unmarried women as well as married women. We are sometimes too quick to divide up into the married/unmarried categories. Though the Bible sometimes singles out different groups, most of the Scriptures address us *all* as God's people, no matter what our individual station.

Galatians 3:28–29 tells us we are "one in Christ Jesus" whether we are male or female, and we are all "heirs according to the promise." We all share the same fundamental duties as Christian people, and our first duty is to worship God rightly. This is of first importance. Paul says to "present your bodies a living sacrifice, holy, acceptable to God, which is your reasonable service" (Rom. 12:1). It is only in light of this most important calling that we should consider the specific duties God lays out for us as women—whether married or not. In other words, our primary calling is to be good Christians. Being a woman is secondary, and being single follows this. In other words, you cannot be a godly single woman if you are not a godly Christian. So we should consider these primary duties first.

This means that you should be giving foremost attention to how you are worshiping God. Are you a woman of prayer? Do you love God's Word? Are you striving to love God with all your heart, soul, mind, and strength? Are you worshiping God on His day in a reverent way that glorifies Him? Are you concerned with obeying Him, no matter what others think or say? Do you love your neighbor? Are you forgiving others? Do you confess your sins? Each of us is called to live a fruitful, obedient, joyful, and abundant life according to the promise. You have a Savior. Your first duty and calling as a Christian is to love and serve Him with a whole heart all your life. This has to be our starting point, because if you are not clear on this, you will not be able to be a fruitful member of His church.

So you need to be in a healthy church, a church that faithfully proclaims the Word, and feeds and shepherds the people. Sometimes people view going to a solid church as just a lucky happenstance rather than the result of a deliberate search. If for some reason you are not in such a church, then you must make every effort to find one, even if it means relocating. In our culture today, Christians relocate for jobs, but seldom for a church.

Actually, the church you are in is far more important than the job you have. If, for some reason, it is entirely impossible for you to be in a good church, then you must be attached to some church, even if it is mediocre. You must be meeting with and worshiping with God's saints. You can still be a woman of the Word and a woman of prayer, even if you don't have a lot of encouragement. Particularly as a single woman, it is very important that you be surrounded by godly, serious Christians who will be a family to you.

After you find a good church, what can you really do as an unmarried woman in the church? Women (whether married or not) are often mentioned in the Bible as helpers, offering support to those who labor with the ministry; they are described as helpers *of the gospel*. In Romans 16, Priscilla (with her husband Aquila) is called a helper (v. 3). The church met in her house. That is no small thing! Mary (v. 6) is described as bestowing much labor on Paul and his band. She must have fed, cared for, and provided housing for Paul and those with him. Phoebe (v. 1) is called a servant of the church. She obviously did so many things for the body of Christ that they were filed in the "too numerous to mention" column. These women are described as serving, sacrificing, bestowing, and helping. Women like this are a tremendous resource in the church. They were in Paul's day, and they still are. But I often think that single women in particular don't realize the huge impact for good they can have in the church. They don't give themselves a good job description, and they don't think they can really be very fruitful (at least in any important manner) until they are having babies. But this is simply false.

2 Peter 1:5–8 gives us all enough to do to keep us very busy for the rest of our lives, insuring that we are fruitful in God's kingdom:

And beside this, giving all diligence, add to your faith virtue; and to virtue knowledge; And to knowledge temperance; and to temperance patience; and to patience godliness; And to godliness brotherly kindness; and to brotherly kindness charity. For if these things be in you, and abound, *they make you that ye shall neither be barren nor unfruitful in the knowledge of our Lord Jesus Christ.* (AV)

I italicized the last part because often unmarried women in particular feel barren and unfruitful because they do not have husbands and children to care for. But look at the wonderful promise in that passage: If we are working hard, paying attention to our spiritual lives, applying ourselves to be more virtuous, godly, kind, charitable, knowledgeable, faithful, patient, and temperate, God promises that we will be far from fruitless. We can be women with fat souls, whether we are married or not.

Single women have many opportunities to be fruitful in their churches. They can find ways to help those who labor in the church. They can be rich in good works, known like Ruth for goodness. Boaz says of Ruth, "For all the people of my town know that you are a virtuous woman" (3:11). Ruth was just looking after her mother-in-law, and the word got out all over town what a good woman she was. Her reputation was connected to her good works. Single women can do all the things the married women can do: they can visit the sick, take a meal to the new mom, take cookies to the Bible study, show hospitality, attend prayer meetings, write a note, or visit the widow. They can get to know the older women and gain wisdom. They can get to know the younger women and encourage them. There is really no limit to what a single woman can do if she is ministry-minded.

I have sometimes told unmarried women to make themselves indispensable, and I have seen them do it. They help out with communion set up or make meals, show hospitality, and help the church in countless ways. And they do this while attending school or working full-time. They are productive members of the church, contributing through much sacrifice and hard work, just like others in the congregation. We need them!

Of course this ministry is not limited to the church. The good works of a single Christian woman should begin with her own immediate family, work out into the church, and overflow into the community. Galatians 6:10 says, "Therefore, as we have opportunity, let us do good to all, especially to those who are of the household of faith." In other words, if you live next door to a widow, by all means reach out to her. Don't think that you should just visit the widows in your church. But God has established the family as our first priority (1 Tim. 5:4, 8) and the church family is next. We should not overlook the needs of our relations because ministering to them is not as glamorous as going into a foreign country to be a missionary. No. God has placed us in families for good reason. We should begin there and love and honor our parents and grandparents first.

Part of the difficulty with all this is the modern mentality of "live for yourself." We are told repeatedly that we deserve this or the other thing. We are encouraged to buy what we want, eat what we want, wear what we want, spend as we want, and do what we want, whenever we want. Unmarried women are targeted especially with this kind of unbiblical propaganda. Christians fall prey to this just like everyone else. I read a Christian book for single women that listed all the advantages of being single. Though it's a great idea to get us all to count our blessings, the author cited all the wrong reasons: married people have to think of someone else all the time, and they can't eat what they want or get up when they want in the morning. Not only is this just an appeal to selfishness, but it turns out to be a cold comfort as well.

Christian women have to live counter-culturally, and this means self-sacrificially. When they begin to give their time and resources to God and serve His people and His church, there are tremendous rewards for everyone: the church is blessed and the one serving others is blessed. And when God is pleased with us, we are most satisfied as His people.

As you begin, or continue, to lay down your life for others, you will find that you do have a place in the church. Your ministry may not be highly visible to everyone, but God sees what you are doing. And those you reach out to will bless God for you. There is nothing that takes our eyes off ourselves and our troubles quite so well as ministering to others who are in need. C. S. Lewis says in one of his letters:

> The pleasure of pride is like the pleasure of scratching. If there is an itch one does want to scratch; but it is much nicer to have neither the itch nor the scratch. As long as we have the itch of self-regard we shall want the pleasure of self-approval; but the happiest moments are those when we forget our precious selves and have neither but have everything else (God, our fellow humans, animals, the garden, and the sky) instead.[1]

Though I believe the single women should be fruitful and helpful in the life of the church, this does not mean that they should shoulder a greater burden than the married women. I certainly don't mean this. Single women have many responsibilities, and they are tired at the end of the day like everyone else. Nevertheless, they should not eliminate themselves from participating in the life of the church, thinking that they will plug in when they are married. We should all be actively looking for ways to love one another throughout our lives. At the same time, we should be realistic. For example, if you don't like babysitting, I'm not saying you are obligated to do it anyway.

1. C. S. Lewis, *Letters of C. S. Lewis* (Houghton Mifflin Harcourt, 2003), 438.

Of course not. But look for opportunities to do the things that you enjoy, and then jump in and participate. This is for your own soul's good, not just everyone else's.

In many evangelical circles, much pressure is put on the single women to go to the mission field. Now of course many women are called and gifted for such things. My mother-in-law served as a missionary in post-war Japan, and she had a fruitful ministry there. My concern is not for women who go to the mission field because they are called, equipped, and eager for it. I bless them! My concern is for the many single women who are manipulated emotionally into going places where they are unprotected, defenseless, and ill-equipped to be. When they struggle with the work, they feel guilty, thinking that if they were really spiritual, they wouldn't mind being so far from home in such a difficult place. It would be far better if they were encouraged from the pulpit to marry, settle down, and raise families.

I've heard evangelical pastors say that if we really want to live sacrificially for Christ, we will volunteer for the mission field. As a general rule, I think unmarried women should not be sent to dangerous frontline missions. Yes, there are always remarkable exceptions to the rule. But just because you have finished your education and are not yet married does not necessarily mean that God wants you to go to the mission field. It's not for everyone. And a seasoned missionary can tell you of many disasters when the wrong people go for the wrong reasons. The mission field is demanding in many ways, and it is difficult enough for married couples to endure the hardships.

So before you consider going, seek counsel, read some missionary biographies, and of course, pray for God's leading.

CHAPTER 4

What About Dad?

One of the big questions that single women often ask is, "What about my dad? How involved should he be in my life?"

This is a question with many angles, depending on your situation. So I am going to try to lay out some basic biblical principles here, and my hope is that you can apply them to your own story.

In a perfect world, we all grow up with loving and sacrificial and protective fathers. Girls always have and always will most definitely need good daddies. But in our imperfect world, things can be and often are very messy. The dads themselves can feel rejected and unnecessary, or unclear of their design and mission. But it's not my job here to go over their responsibilities; rather, I'm going to go over the responsibilities of daughters.

The first principle is laid out in Ephesians 6:1-3: "Children, obey your parents in the Lord, for this is right. 'Honor your father and mother,' which is the first commandment with promise: 'that it may be well with you and you may live long on the earth.'"

Are you a daughter? Do you have parents? Then you are required to obey them when you are a child, and you are required to honor them all your days. But when does obedience cease to be required? I believe that strict obedience is no longer required when a daughter is no longer under her parents' roof and is providing for herself. In other words, if your dad is paying your rent and your tuition, you should still strive to obey him. Hopefully, as you've grown up, he doesn't really need to give you any "commands" anymore like he did when you were a toddler. And if you were an obedient daughter when you were young, you probably didn't need much supervision once you hit the double digits. But some girls are rebellious and disrespectful all the way up. If that describes you, then the first order of business is to put some things right. Were you sneaking out when your parents wanted you home? Stealing money from your mom's purse? Lying about where you had been? If so, then it is never too late to apologize to them and ask for their forgiveness. Put things right on your side as far as is possible with you.

But if you are a daughter who has always enjoyed a happy relationship with your parents, then you are blessed indeed. Don't take that for granted! My point here is that the goal of childrearing is to get the children to internalize the Christian standards their parents are teaching them. But if your parents were letting you figure things out on your own, or teaching you ungodly standards, you should thank God that He picks you up where you are and not where you should have been.

At some point then, your parents have ceased to require obedience. If they are still giving you commands when you are in your mid-twenties and self-supporting, then you may need to find some help to disentangle yourself.

So much for the command to obey your parents. Once you are an adult (and by that I mean no longer relying on their support), you should continue to honor your parents as much as possible. This means that you are courteous, deferential, kind, and hold them in reverence. You honor the position they hold as your parents, even if you disagree with how they are living.

God really likes it when we honor our parents. In fact, He has added a promise to this commandment. By honoring our parents, our lives will go better. We will live longer. We will be blessed ("it will go well with you"). Therefore, we should be eager to honor our parents. What if your parents are not living? In that case, you can honor their memory. You can share good stories about them and recount the ways you admired them. You do not have to share their failures and sins.

Whatever kind of parents (or parent) God gave us, we should thank Him for them, and we should pray for them as long as they live. In fact, we may be called to care for them in their old age. This is part of God's plan for children and parents. So prepare for that by stewarding your relationship with them now.

How much authority should a dad (in particular) or parents have when it comes to the man you want to marry? If you are living at home, Dad is still the head of the home. You should seek his input when it comes to guys, and you should introduce him as soon as possible to any young men who come around. He understands young men much better than you do! And of course, your mom should not be left out of this process. Hopefully, you have discussed dating and courtship with your parents and you already know what they expect.

I grew up in a home where I had a good relationship with my parents. They set the curfew for my dates, but they didn't say much more about it. In fact, when Doug and I got engaged, I called my parents to let them know. Their response was, "To whom, honey?" That was not because I was disobedient or disrespectful. It was simply the way I had grown up. After my parents were married in the early 1940's, they drove across the country so my mom could meet her in-laws!

That was not the way we brought our children up. We wanted to be much more involved in the process. So if you don't know your parents' thoughts and expectations, you should check in. They may be more like my parents (whatever you want, honey) or they may be more like us, where Doug told the girls to send any interested guys to him. They loved that arrangement because they could either say no thanks themselves, or they could hand it off to their Dad, and he handled it for them. Once they found "the one," Doug set the boundaries and checked in often to see how things were going along. It worked beautifully, thank the Lord.

But what if your dad is not a believer? In that case, don't try to get him to act like one. He can't. And it will only annoy him and frustrate you. If he is not interested in getting to know a man whom you are interested in, don't force it. God has given you the dad you have, so be grateful. If you must navigate this alone, then ask God for wisdom, and proceed with caution and prayer. But don't resent your parents.

If you succeed in forcing your parents to get involved, you may regret their involvement after all. So just work with what God has given you. If you have been out of the home for years, supporting yourself, you are still required to honor your parents, and that means keeping them in the loop. If you met a great guy, let them know. Don't ask them for advice unless you really want it. But if you do, then by all means, ask away. Just realize that asking them for their advice puts you in the position of having to decide if you agree or disagree. And if you won't follow their advice anyway, why complicate your life?

Treasure your parents. Respect your dad. Love your mom. Maintain a good relationship if you have one. Pray for a better relationship if you don't have a good one. Practice telling your dad how you respect him by focusing on his abilities and achievements. Practice telling your mom how much you love her and appreciate her sacrifice and support. You will get better at it. And if you happen to have a wonderful relationship with godly parents, then you are blessed indeed. Don't squander it or take it for granted. Tell them how blessed you are, and enjoy this good gift from God.

CHAPTER 5

Is This Really God's Best?

Good doctrine protects us from all kinds of errors and all kinds of fears. One of the important things you must know, understand, and *believe* is that God has planned good for you and not evil. He loves His children. His providence rules His world, and He governs His people with kindness. "All the paths of the Lord are mercy and truth, to such as keep His covenant and His testimonies" (Ps. 25:10). If you have a solid, biblical doctrine, not only of God's sovereignty, but also of His wisdom and love for you, this will protect you from many doubts, worries, and fears about the future, as well as keep you from fretting over the past.

Years ago, a young woman asked me what I thought about her praying for a husband. She had been taught that God didn't know the future, so He didn't know whether she would marry or not. This made her wonder what the point of praying could be. Bad doctrine has bad consequences. Good doctrine teaches us to ask God for the good things He created. He mandated marriage; it was His idea. So a Christian woman should be able to ask God to bestow His good gift of marriage on her. I have sometimes told women to "tug on the Lord's sleeve." He likes us to persevere in prayer!

In the meantime, she can expect to be assailed with temptations to worry about the future: What if I never marry? What if I marry, but it is too late to have children? What if there is no one for me after all? What if I missed "God's best"? These are questions that are impossible to answer because all "what if" questions are not really questions at all, but doubts. They disrupt your peace and bring troubling thoughts; they rob you of your joy by introducing fictional and future trials. Jesus warned us not to borrow trouble because each day has enough of its own (Mt. 6:34). These sorts of thoughts are temptations, and God wants you to learn to deal with temptations, whatever form they take.

Jesus tells us not to be anxious about our lives (Mt. 6:31–33). We are to cast all our cares on Him because He cares for us (1 Pet. 5:7). Worrying will only make life miserable. It is fruitless. It is telling ourselves bad stories. So how should you deal with temptations that come in the form of "what if" questions? This may seem like a simplistic answer, but here it is: ignore them. Do not answer them; in fact, do not listen to them. Rather, ask what good things God has given you to do today. Focus on today's duties. This is a fruitful use of your time. Recognize that those "what if" questions are temptations to get you to feel blue, worried, lonely, or anxious. Do not engage in a conversation with yourself about this stuff. Ignore, ignore, ignore. And set your mind on something helpful, something that is profitable. This is how we fear God. And when we fear God, that holy fear swallows up all our other petty fears.

If you have a long history of worrying about such things, it may take you a while to change your habits. You may not even realize how much time each day you are thinking such thoughts. Start paying attention to your thought habits and reject the questions. Do not listen. If you were listening to a playlist of obnoxious music, you would change it. Do the same thing with the conversation in your mind. Change it!

Jesus has promised that He will *never leave you* or forsake you (Heb. 13:5). This is the reason that every Christian can be content with the circumstances God has given. He is always with us through every trial. I will deal more directly with contentment in chapter six. Thomas Watson, the great Puritan preacher, wrote that "It is our work to cast away care; and it is God's work to take care."[1] God's Word is full of promises to us, so let's believe them and rest in God's care for us.

Another harassing temptation that can assault an unmarried woman is to fret over the past. "Maybe I should have married so-and-so after all." "I wonder if I was being too picky . . ." "Maybe I should have gone on that singles' retreat . . ." Notice that temptations about the future often begin with "What if," but temptations about the past often begin with "Maybe I should have . . ." or "I wonder if . . ." And of course, these have no legitimate answer either. The only way to respond to "What if I never get married?" is to say, "What if I do?" And the only way to answer, "Maybe I should have married Steve" is to say "Maybe I shouldn't have!" Some wise saint has said, "Don't doubt in the dark what you knew in the light." If it was clear that Steve was not the one back "in the light of day," don't begin to worry about it now. You may be feeling lonely, and that has affected your good judgment. Once you get into a worrying state of mind, you have a low sales resistance to other sins: self-pity, bitterness, self-centeredness, and so forth.

If you have sinned objectively, confess it. For example, if you knew that Steve was a godly man that you respected highly, but you didn't want to give up your non-Christian boyfriend, then that is certainly an objective sin to confess. But doubts don't go away, even if you confess them all day long, because you are

1. Thomas Watson, *The Art of Divine Contentment* (Glasgow: Free Presbyterian Publications, n.d.).

confessing the wrong thing. Don't confess the doubts; rather, confess listening to the doubts, and then forsake the wrong doing. Quit listening! Don't fret about the past and don't worry about the future.

Have you ever noticed how unattractive worry is on other people? Being anxiety-ridden is like taking ugly pills. This kind of worry is really self-centeredness. Being self-absorbed and worrisome is about keeping me and my life and my future all on center stage. On the other hand, a spirit that is resting in the Lord and rejoicing in Him is lovely to behold. This kind of spirit can focus on others and is not distracted with its own needs. Cultivate this kind of internal beauty and quit taking the ugly pills.

As you get rid of worry of all kinds, replace it with the right kind of thinking. You are not living out God's second best. He is writing your story, and it is a good one. Believe Him. If you are walking in faith, you have grounds to believe that your story is a blessed one. But if you are living in disobedience, you may think you need to take the pen to write the next chapter yourself. You might be afraid of what God has in store for you. But He promises blessing to those who walk in His covenant. If you are living in disobedience, then you have no grounds for assuming that the story has a happy ending. But if you are walking by faith, confessing your sins, and seeking to please God, you can know that He will bless you. Your faith may be tested, but so is everyone's. Remember that testing produces patience, experience, and hope (Rom. 5:3–5, AV). God tailors our circumstances according to our soul's needs, for our soul's good. This should be a source of comfort to us. God is concerned with the health of our souls, and we should think the same way He does.

God's promises are not just for the married people. They are for all those who are His. Your duty is to believe Him. Believe that He is ordering your life for your good and His glory. Then look around to your duties so you can serve Him more devotedly, more entirely, more fully. Ask Him to give you great joy in your duties as you trust Him. Refuse to play any guessing games or "what if" games that destroy your joy and trouble your soul. You can then be sure that not only is your life *not* God's second-best plan for you, but that it is the abundant life that Christ promised, a life that is full of peace and overflowing with joy.

Asking God for a husband is a good thing. Persevere in it. Continue to remind Him that you want to be married. Tug on His sleeve. But don't fret over it. As you pray, do all in your power to "make it happen," without compromising your biblical standards. But we will address the things that you can do in later chapters.

CHAPTER 6

Don't Be a Basket Case

In the last chapter I mentioned that when women worry, it is as though they are taking ugly pills. All sin of every kind is destructive, but some sin really can work itself out onto a woman's countenance making her visibly unattractive. Anxiety and bitterness are like that. A peaceful woman, with a gentle and quiet spirit, grows more and more beautiful from the inside out; but a woman with a discontented spirit gets uglier and uglier.

Today it is almost expected that you will have "issues," be depressed, or come from a "dysfunctional" family. Real troubles have real biblical solutions, though some may be very difficult. But some women find security in *having* hang-ups and troubles. It gives them a story and provides an identity for them. But we should find our identity in Christ. He has freed us from our sins. He has written, and is writing, a much better and more beautiful story. Yes, we all have troubles. Everyone has troubles. But you can determine to get help for your troubles so you can press on in your Christian life, and not drag your family's sins or your own messed up past (or present) with you into the future.

How do you do this? Of course the specifics will vary with each woman, but here are a few starting principles. First, take a look at your shortcomings. What are they? If you were a character in a book you were reading, would you like the character? If not, why? What sort of transformation needs to take place? What does the Bible say about your situation? God's Word addresses everything. Are you reading your Bible regularly? You may need to seek forgiveness from your parents, a friend, a teacher, or a boss. You may need to pay old debts off, return stolen goods, or confess to cheating on a test. This is simply taking care of business.

If you need help, go to your pastor and get his advice and counsel on how to proceed. The important thing here is that you are making every effort to progress in your Christian walk and not putting things off. We all underestimate the polluting effects of sin in our lives. Putting your affection on Christ means putting off things like sexual impurity, anger, lying, covetousness, and filthy talk (Col. 3:1-10). All of us, married or single, cannot afford to be complacent about sin. Even if you have managed to camouflage some of your sin so that your friends don't see it, you cannot hide it from God. Deal with it all by the grace of God.

Sin is a weight and a hindrance and needs to be confessed and forsaken. But how do you deal with all your family's issues? First of all, you have to sort out which, if any, of these problems is actually your responsibility. Your parents' marriage, for example, is not your responsibility to fix. On the other hand, if your behavior has made things difficult for them, you must seek their forgiveness. But you cannot confess their sins or make their troubles go away. You need to cast your cares on the Lord and not try to shoulder them yourself. You can't carry it, and you can't fix it. But you can pray, and you can ask God to bring help. You must quit feeling like it is all your responsibility.

The same is true of your siblings' troubles. Yes, we are to bear one another's burdens, but we must remember what that means. It includes prayer, offering counsel, support, and encouragement. But as you come along side them to offer these things, you must keep your perspective. This is your sister or brother, not your son or daughter. Women can feel an awful burden of responsibility for things that are someone else's responsibility. So remember your place and offer help without making other people's problems your own. This will actually make you more effective in helping them, not less. And though the world has found a certain kind of glamour in having lots of horrible problems, or coming from a family that does, the Christian has found life and grace in Christ where all the sin is dealt with.

My dear mother-in-law came from a family with lots of troubles. When she was five, her mother died suddenly, and her father took a job a couple hundred miles away. That left her older siblings to care for her. But I had known her some years before I ever heard about some of the hardships of her childhood, growing up without her parents. When she finally told me about some of these things, it was in the context of how blessed my own children were. It was not a sob story or a self-pity party. She was living in the resurrection. God had delivered her out of her past, and He had given her many opportunities to minister to her family members over the years. She did not live in defeat; nor did she glory in the sins of her family. She had gone on to live a productive, fruitful Christian life. This is what we all must do.

Bad habits can also make us ineffective and unattractive. Though not all bad habits are sins in themselves, they are always ugly, and most of them spring from some sin or other, even if the thing itself seems to be neutral.

What kinds of things do I mean? Nervous habits like nail-biting may spring from anxiety or tension, and though God does not forbid chewing on your nails, He does forbid anxiety. Everyone agrees that these are not pretty habits. Bad lifestyle habits like smoking, overeating, drinking too much, over-spending, or bad housekeeping are not beautifying. They do not adorn the Christian woman but rather hold her back and hinder her progress. These things can all be overcome, and some take more time than others to gain victory over. The first step is to identify the area that needs to be sanctified. Then help can be sought out if necessary and the plan of attack can be laid out.

Cultivate beautifying habits and determine to pitch the ugly ones overboard. You will be happier, and you will be encour-aged to press on in your Christian life with fewer hindrances holding you back. It is amazing how much these "little" things really can weigh a woman down.

Don't think these kinds of bad habits will be easier to deal with later. You certainly don't want to take them with you into a marriage, and you don't want to carry them with you the rest of your unmarried life. Either way, you want to press on in Christ and decide to have "no issues" as far as it is possible with you.

When a man is considering marriage, he has to determine whether he will be able to shoulder the responsibility of a wife. A wife who is bogged down with her own troubles will be a great weight; and a wife who is already thriving spiritually will be a positive help. A woman wants to prepare herself to be a help to a man, not a project for him to take on. So press on in your Christian life. Be diligent to pursue godliness. Grow in grace!

CHAPTER 7

Don't Pretend to Be Happy

One of the many temptations for unmarried women is to pretend to be happy. Now before you throw this book across the room, let me explain. I think that unmarried women *should* be happy, of course, and I know many who are. Contentment is required of us all, and unmarried women have much to be thankful for.

But here is the temptation: if you are struggling with contentment, longing to be married, and not always being thankful for your unmarried state, it is easy to want to hide it from everyone else. If you admit that you want to be married, you may think (wrongly) that you are admitting a weakness or a fault. Or you might not want to seem like a marriage nerd, always on the lookout for "him." So you pretend to be doing fine when, in fact, you are *not* doing fine. You may even convince yourself (while dogmatically telling others) that you don't really want marriage right now, that you're not interested in a relationship because you don't have the time. But we all know that if God sent the right man along right now, you would happily drop everything in a heartbeat. And we would commend you for it.

Imagine a conversation with a sweet Christian woman who is in this kind of jam. You run into her and ask how she is doing. She then falls all over herself telling you how much she loves her job, how busy she is, how much traveling she is doing, how she really doesn't have any time (or need) for a social life. Or she tells you about her classes, when she'll have her degree, and all the wonderful job possibilities waiting out there for her. Now I'm *certainly not* saying that she is lying about all this. Don't get me wrong here. But I *am* saying that it is *possible* that this is all just a very hollow cover to make you think she is "happy, happy, happy all the day" when she would really like to cry and say she hates all of this. She might really want to tell you that she is miserable, frustrated, and lonely traveling by herself, that she wishes she could be doing something that would give her more fulfillment and make her feel more a part of the body of Christ. But this, she thinks, would be admitting defeat, and so she convinces herself that her career is all she wants after all.

Part of the way to freedom for women in this bind is to help them see, first of all, that it is not only okay, but positively healthy to want to be married. There is nothing in the world wrong with wanting to be married. It is only wrong to be miserable about it. And wanting to be married does not equal discontent. Many women are feeling a false guilt about this. It goes something like this: "If I were truly godly, I wouldn't want to be married. I would be happy to be unmarried for the rest of my life. But I do long to be married, therefore I am not rejoicing in the Lord, and therefore I am guilty of sin." But you can confess false guilt all day long and never feel forgiven. God forgives real sin not our imagined sin.

God created marriage, and He has given women a desire for marriage. This is good. I suggest that an unmarried woman thank God that she longs to be married. Thank Him that He has given you these desires, and ask Him to keep you and protect you in them. He wants to take up our burdens, so you can ask Him to bear the burden of your longing for marriage. He will do it. This requires faith and courage: faith that God will do what He says, and courage to walk with Him through this time. Each of us needs faith and courage if we want to please God, so rejoice in the opportunity He is giving you to grow in both these areas.

And God does not disapprove of His children wanting things. He invites us to ask Him for good things, and marriage is a good thing. We simply must remember in all of life that we are to cultivate gratitude and contentment, knowing God rules the world, He loves His children, and He delights to give us good things. We may ask God for marriage, but we must do it with gratitude in our hearts.

> Be anxious for nothing, but in everything by prayer and supplication, with thanksgiving, let your requests be made known to God; and the peace of God, which surpasses all understanding, will guard your hearts and minds through Christ Jesus. (Phil. 4:6–7)

This is a spectacular promise. We are to be careful for nothing. *No thing.* In fact, Peter tells us we are to cast all our cares on Him because He cares for us (1 Pet. 5:7). But the verse right before is important in understanding *how* we cast our cares: "Therefore humble yourselves under the mighty hand of God, that he may exalt you in due time." We bow and submit ourselves under God's mighty hand, and He lifts us up in His perfect time. We throw all our cares on Him, and He carries them for us. He is obviously far more capable of carrying them than we are anyway. Jesus said,

> Come to Me, all you who labor and are heavy laden, and
> I will give you rest. Take My yoke upon you and learn

from Me, for I am gentle and lowly in heart, and you will find rest for your souls. For My yoke is easy and My burden is light. (Mt. 11:28–30)

We come to Christ in prayer with all our cares and longings. And we make our requests to Him with thanksgiving. We thank Him for His care for us, for His love for us. We lay our burdens down at His feet, and He promises rest for our souls, and peace of heart and mind. That is an easy yoke. And what a trade off: we give Him our cares and He gives our souls rest. These are promises for all of us, for the married and unmarried alike.

An unmarried woman can come to Christ in prayer with all her requests, but she must do it with thanksgiving. Of course she cannot be thankful if she thinks it is sinful for her to keep asking for marriage over and over. But if she realizes that it is not a sinful desire after all, she can ask with joy, anticipation, and thankfulness, living without anxiety because she has found peace and rest in Christ. She doesn't cease to desire marriage and children. But she does quit faking it because now she *really is* happy. By confessing the *right* sins, she can start anew.

So you'd like to be married? Good. Don't worry about it. And don't worry about worrying about it. Do you have a great job? Good. Rejoice that God has given you good things to do. Are you in school? Good. Study hard. Are you lonely sometimes? Don't worry about that either. Loneliness is not a sin.

This kind of contented attitude is only possible if you are deliberately taking on the easy yoke of Christ and learning from Him, our meek and lowly Savior. Jeremiah Burroughs, in his wonderful book *The Rare Jewel of Christian Contentment*, defines contentment this way: "Christian contentment is that sweet, inward, quiet, gracious frame of spirit, which freely submits to and delights in God's wise and fatherly disposal in

1. Jeremiah Burroughs, *The Rare Jewel of Christian Contentment* (Edinburgh: Banner of Truth, 2005).

every condition."[1] This is victorious Christian living. He also points out that when we are troubled by our circumstances, we should listen to the grace of contentment speaking to us: "O under, under! Get you under, O soul! Keep under! Keep low! Keep under God's feet! You are under God's feet, and keep under his feet! Keep under the authority of God, the majesty of God, the sovereignty of God, the power that God has over you! To keep under, that is to submit."[2] And, I would add, to be under God is the only safe place, and surely it is the only place where contentment is possible.

Without this humble attitude of contentment, it is easy to become unhappy, and then there is a host of other temptations. One of these is to look for happiness in all the wrong places. For example, if a woman has a job that she likes, it is possible for her to throw herself into it for the wrong reason, and that wrong reason is that she is trying to find meaning, identity, purpose, and happiness in her job because she thinks that will keep her from being sad over not being married. But as we've seen above, the only thing that keeps us all from being sad in any kind of hard circumstance is contentment in Christ. A job won't meet our emotional and spiritual needs, no matter how great a job it is. If you pour yourself into "ministry" in the church, expecting that to "meet your needs," then you will be sorely disappointed. These things are not designed by God to satisfy our souls in that way. Again, only Christ can put us right. For that matter, marriage won't satisfy us either. Any time we look to a created thing to do what only the Creator can do, we are guilty of idolatry. Marriage is a created thing, and it is good. It is a means of glorifying God; it is not an end in itself.

Learning to be content while you are unmarried is a terrific advantage. Married women struggle with contentment like ev-

2. Ibid.

eryone else, so if you have learned to do this now, you will be able to apply it your whole life. And I believe that if you are a discontented unmarried woman, you will certainly be a discontented married woman. Marriage simply amplifies all that we are; it doesn't change our nature. Just turns up the volume. If you are prone to be self-centered while you are unmarried, marriage will just increase your opportunities to demonstrate this kind of selfishness. That is why you should determine to learn contentment before you are married; otherwise you are just postponing the lesson. The book of Proverbs has a few things to say about the state of a man who lives with a discontented woman: it would be better for him to live in a corner on the roof than in a big house with a brawling woman (21:9); living with a contentious woman is like putting up with a constant dripping; a man would be happier living out in the woods or in the desert than with a cantankerous woman (21:19).

Paul says he has *learned* contentment. If the great apostle had to learn this lesson, so must we. It does not come naturally to us. Let me quote this section from Philippians 4:11–13:

> Not that I speak in regard to need, for I have learned in whatever state I am, to be content: I know how to be abased, and I know how to abound. Everywhere and in all things I have learned both to be full and to be hungry, both to abound and to suffer need. I can do all things through Christ who strengthens me.

Notice that Paul has learned to be content in all kinds of circumstances. He sometimes had all that he needed and more; and at other times he suffered great need. How did he manage to be content through all this? Christ enabled and strengthened him. This famous verse "I can do all things through Christ who strengthens me" appears in the context of a discussion about contentment. That is the key to being contented women:

looking to Christ who strengthens us. That is the promise. We cannot look to ourselves to find contentment. That would be profoundly discouraging. We cannot look to our circumstances as the source of contentment. They change too much. But God is the same yesterday, today, and forever. He never leaves us or forsakes us. He carries our burdens and leads us through all kinds of circumstances, whether it is in times of plenty or times of want. It is okay for an unmarried woman to identify with the "want." She does not have to pretend that she is ambivalent toward marriage. I think that half the battle in learning contentment is recognizing where we are "in want" so that we can effectively deal with it.

Burroughs suggests in his book that instead of trying to get our circumstances up to match our desires, and therefore finding contentment, we should instead be striving to get our desires down to match our circumstances. What this means is that the unmarried woman seeks to be satisfied with God in her life now, while asking Him to provide a husband in the future. She doesn't have to quit "desiring" marriage; rather, she must have an equally great desire to rejoice in the Lord now.

One of the ways the single woman can guard against discontent is to closely oversee her thought life. She must guard against envying couples and not allow herself to indulge in unkind or ungrateful thoughts about any of her sisters or brothers in Christ. (This would include thinking that "He must be crazy to go for a girl like her.") She must not be resentful when a close friend gets engaged, but rejoice with those who rejoice. She must reject the temptations to jealousy and competition. If an eligible man befriends several women in the same group of friends, they each must keep from developing a competitive spirit. The contented spirit is in a better position to reject all these temptations to ungodliness, but a woman who is already discontent will be drawn more easily into these other sins. Bur-

3. Ibid.

roughs says, "The devil loves to fish in troubled waters."[3] In other words, a woman who already has a bad attitude (discontent) will be an easy target when it comes to other sinful attitudes. But once discontent is dealt with, other sins will be more readily identified and temptations more easily resisted.

Of course, once we attain contentment in one situation, we most certainly will be tempted to become discontent again, either over the same issue or over a different one. This is a lifelong struggle called our sanctification. We must remember that, "He who has begun a good work in you will complete it until the day of Jesus Christ" (Phil. 1:6). Chapter four of Deuteronomy enjoins us to "take heed to thyself, and keep thy soul diligently" (v. 9, AV). Later in the same chapter we are reminded again to "take heed to yourselves" (v. 23) and "take careful heed to yourselves" (v. 15). Why do we take heed of our souls? "Lest you forget the covenant of the LORD your God" (v. 23). We all must take care to watch ourselves and take heed or pay attention to the state of our souls. How are we really doing? The unmarried woman must not kid herself about how she is doing. If she is happily unmarried and trusting God for her future, she is able to be a productive, fruitful member of the church community. She is free from thinking hard thoughts about God herself and asking why God is doing this "to me." And she realizes God is not doing this *to* her, but *for* her. Then she can enjoy God's people without bitterness or envy.

A discontented woman is also very vulnerable when it comes to receiving attention from men that she knows full well are wrong for her. She rationalizes. If she is longing to be married and has an impatient, discontented heart, she will be more likely to consider someone who will make her far unhappier than she is now. A contented heart clears the mind and protects good judgment. A woman who has been thinking of nothing but "marriage at any cost," will be more likely to respond to the first man who comes along, even if he is entirely unsuitable.

There is one thing worse than not being married, and that is being married to the wrong guy. I have spoken with a number of unhappy wives over the years, and I have asked many of them, "Why did you marry him?" Some women confess that they knew it was unwise at the time, but they went forward with it anyway. Don't make such a costly mistake.

One of the best antidotes to keep discontent away is to cultivate a spirit of gratitude. We are to be a grateful people:

> Enter into His gates with thanksgiving, and into His courts with praise. Be thankful to Him, and bless His name. For the LORD is good; His mercy is everlasting, and His truth endures to all generations. (Ps. 100:4–5)

The unmarried woman should adorn herself with gratitude to God for everything all the time. Yes, this requires grace from God, but He loves to bestow His grace upon us. He always enables us to do what He requires. He commands us to be full of gratitude: "And whatever you do in word or deed, do all in the name of the Lord Jesus, giving thanks to God the Father through Him" (Col. 3:17). Spurgeon uses this example in teaching on contentment: "I have heard of some good old woman in a cottage, who had nothing but a piece of bread and a little water. Lifting up her hands, she said as a blessing, 'What! All this, and Christ too?'"[4] But if you think, "I cannot thank Him for my unmarried state. I will thank Him for my job or the weather, but I will not thank Him for that," then you have identified your root problem. Confess to God your lack of thankfulness for all things, including the fact that you are not married, and ask Him to give you a spirit of gratitude, thanksgiving, and rejoicing in all things. "Rejoice in the Lord

---

4. *Sermons Delivered in Exter Hall, Strand, During the Enlargement of New Park* (London: Alabaster & Passmore, 1855), 89.

always. Again I will say, rejoice!" (Phil. 4:4). You are where you are on purpose. He knows what He is doing. This is not "Plan B." Submit to His good plans for you and thank Him for all He is doing. Then you will be in a position to ask for more. Yes, this takes faith, but that is what being a Christian is about: walking by faith in a good and holy God. This is living a grace-filled life.

CHAPTER 8

Cheerfulness is Good Medicine

Connected to contentment is the virtue of cheerfulness. God makes much of this, especially considering Scripture's many positive admonitions to cheerfulness and negative images associated with the dismal lack of cheeriness. Sometimes the single woman has trouble reconciling her desire to be married with a cheerful happiness in her circumstances. If she really longs to be married, how can she live in a happy, cheerful manner? Wouldn't that be to deny her desire for something else? No, these things are not mutually exclusive. A woman can have a deep desire for a husband and still rejoice before the Lord in the circumstances He has ordained for her. And she does not have to confess her desire for marriage as sin. It isn't. But discontentment and a grumbling attitude are sins. She should determine to be cheerful in her unmarried state while she longs and prays for a husband, because this is pleasing to God. And, besides, a cheerful woman is far more appealing to a Christian man than a discontented woman.

The Christian woman, no matter what her state, has a duty to be cheerful. The single woman, because of temptations to loneliness, self-pity, or discontent, must determine to be cheerful and helpful, wise and grateful to God. The last thing she really wants is to have people feeling sorry for her. And a lack of cheerfulness is a character flaw; it is not based on circumstances. If a single woman is glum, she will certainly take that glumness with her into marriage. Even if she thinks the reason for her sadness is because she is single, after marriage she will find new reasons to be unhappy. We are to rejoice *in the Lord,* not in our circumstances. Our reason for cheerfulness is found in Him, not in any situation or creature.

In other words, for every Christian, the *source* of our happiness is God, and the *direction* of our happiness is toward Him as well. He bestows a spirit of joy upon us, and we return it to Him in our praise and thanksgiving. The unmarried woman must make use of God's grace to walk in a spirit of joy and cheerfulness, paying attention to her demeanor and conduct, striving to please God and to be a source of comfort and blessing to those around her. This is a basic duty for all Christians, not just for those women without the joys of a husband and children. It would be easy to slip into a negative mindset, and this is unhealthy, unbiblical, undisciplined, and unattractive. A cheerful attitude is a grace that bestows loveliness. And Proverbs says that a merry heart is good medicine (17:22). When we adopt a cheerful demeanor, we cheer ourselves up as well as those around us.

When Jesus healed the paralytic in Matthew 9, He said, "Son, be of good cheer; your sins are forgiven you" (v. 2). Having our sins forgiven is a tremendous reason to be cheerful. A clean conscience, to be washed, restored, and put right with God is an immeasurable blessing. But sometimes Christians begin to get accustomed to the idea that they are a forgiven people, and they take it for granted. Then they become complacent in their joy, and they allow discontentment to creep in. Women must be particularly prone to the sin of grumbling, because Proverbs describes the woman whose husband would rather live in a corner of the roof than be around her constant complaining (21:9). She is compared to a leaky, drippy faucet, nagging and griping in a nonstop, monotonous fashion (27:15). This must get under control before marriage, because married life has many provocations of its own.

In his commentary on Proverbs, Charles Bridges describes the plight of the man married to the woman who is a "continual dropping on a very rainy day" (27:15–16): "There is rain without and within, both alike troublesome; the one preventing us from going abroad with comfort; the other from staying at home in peace. The storm within is however much the most pitiless. Shelter may be found from the other. None from this."[1]

Scripture tells us to give cheerfully (2 Cor. 9:7); to show mercy with cheerfulness (Rom. 12:8); and to sing psalms as an outlet for our cheerfulness (Jas. 5:13). Apparently, showing mercy and giving financially are two areas of particular temptation. The third area is hospitality: "Use hospitality one to another without grudging" (1 Pet. 4:9, AV). A good dose of cheerfulness will deal with this. Our cheerfulness should have direction, as stated before. We should express this by singing, giving, and praising God. All these things (mercy, giving, and hospitality) are particularly in women's domain: bringing up children, lodging strangers, washing the saints' feet, relieving the afflicted, and diligently following every good work. These activities are listed in 1 Timothy 5 as qualifying an older widow to receive church support. So it is safe to say these things lie in women's domain. In all these things there are many temptations to lose our cheerfulness.

Christian women, whether married or not, should cultivate a spirit of cheeriness when showing mercy. Whether she is extending forgiveness to someone who has wronged her or

---

1. Charles Bridges, *Proverbs* (Edinburgh: Banner of Truth Trust, 1994), 515.

bestowing pity and compassion on someone who is in need, all should be done in good spirits, with pleasantness and brightness. When giving financially, it should not be given out of a guilty conscience or with second thoughts. God loves it when we give happily and cheerfully. When showing hospitality (planned or unplanned), it is good to remember our sister Martha and not give way to a grumpy attitude when we find ourselves alone in the kitchen with no helpers. Rather than a long face, or with a begrudging spirit, let it be done with joy.

Psalms and Proverbs have many verses describing the happiness of those who are blessed, and single women have access to these very same blessings. Consider just these few.

> *Blessed* is every one who fears the LORD, who walks in His ways. When you eat the labor of your hands, you shall be *happy*, and it shall be well with you. (Ps. 128:1–2)

> *Happy* is the man who finds wisdom, and the man who gains understanding. (Prov. 3:13)

> He who heeds the word wisely will find *good*, and whoever trusts in the LORD, *happy* is he. (Prov. 16:20)

> Where there is no revelation, the people cast off restraint; but *happy* is he who keeps the law. (Prov. 29:18)

> *Happy* are the people whose God is the LORD!
> (Ps. 144:15b)

Look at the verbs in these verses: *fears, walks, finds, gains, heeds, trusts, keeps.* Now look a little closer: fears *the Lord*, walks *in His ways*, finds *wisdom*, gains *understanding*, heeds *the word*, trusts *the Lord*, and keeps *the law*.

God brings us blessing and happiness (and cheerfulness) when we give ourselves to Him. When we walk in the fear of the Lord, obeying His Word, worshiping with His saints, faithfully applying all we learn, we can look for the joy, blessedness, and happiness that attend those who live this way. God is faithful and He will do this. When we are trusting Him and rejoicing in the Lord, it is much harder to give ourselves over to anxiety or murmuring and complaining.

Those things which hinder cheerfulness (like unbelief, impatience, and ingratitude) cannot survive in a climate of trust and law-keeping. As we do all things to His glory, giving thanks as we go, the Spirit stirs us up to more love for God. This in turn makes us more fruitful and thankful, charitable and compassionate, cheerful and tender.

The Christian woman who has these graces is far more appealing, attractive, and fun to be with. Rather than living in misery and sadness, a woman who has a bright spirit of cheerfulness has a more blessed existence. She is too busy thinking of how to please God to be glum about her own circumstances.

CHAPTER 9

Dressing with a Worldview

The term *modesty* frequently conjures up ideas of sunbonnets, calico dresses, and odd swimwear. But modesty for the modern Christian woman does not need to look like the modesty of centuries past. We need to get beyond some of our stereotypical ideas of what biblical modesty is like so we can get a handle on dressing in a manner that is consistent with our identity in Christ.

While we emphasize Christian worldview thinking in many areas like literature, politics, the arts, and science, some of the most obvious everyday applications get overlooked. This is all part of our sanctification: we are still learning to spread our love of Christ into every realm of our lives. Meanwhile, one of these neglected areas of application is women's clothing. Though there seems to be plenty of teaching on modesty, somehow many Christian women still don't see the connection between loving God with all our heart, soul, mind, and strength and getting dressed in the morning.

Let's adopt the biblical terms of *wise* and *foolish* in this discussion of modesty. After all, a woman who is wise will dress wisely, and the foolish woman dresses like a fool. But there is also a third category, and that is the *naïve* or *simple* woman. These women and their characteristics are described for us in Proverbs, so let's consider how each applies her worldview when it comes to dressing.

First, consider the naïve or simple woman. She should know better, but she doesn't. She may have been listening, but she doesn't *do* what she hears, so she really doesn't get it. She is like the silly women in 2 Timothy (3:6–7) who are always learning but never coming to an understanding of the truth. When she hears good teaching, she will tone it down, explain it away, or apply it to other people. She is easily swayed, easily impressed, cares too much what people think of her (the wrong kind of people, that is), and she underestimates the dangers of her behavior. She is culturally immature, and this may show up in the form of a little butterfly tattoo, a strand of purple hair, or a nose stud, or it may manifest itself in her dress when she wears a jumper two sizes too big. She might be the kind who will refuse to wear makeup and leave her hair uncut, unstyled, uncombed, and unkempt. Or she may be a bubble-gum chewing airhead who wears dumb T-shirts and can't figure out why the guys keep staring at her chest. The naïve woman needs to take heed to wisdom. It is time for her to grow up, to take responsibility for her behavior, and accept wisdom. She can be easily persuaded to follow, and if she has wise friends, she may be led into wisdom herself.

The foolish woman knows nothing. She is without discretion, easily flattered, vain, self-centered, and she will not receive correction. Her inappropriate dress or behavior is "her own business," and she enjoys the impact it is having on the men. If they stare at her, she flatters herself. If someone tries to talk with her about modesty, she gets prickly and offended or attributes the correction to jealousy or envy. She foolishly assumes she knows more than those who are older or wiser, whether it is her parents, her teacher, her boss, a friend, or her pastor. This woman is the kind that mothers warn their sons about.

Unfortunately, the foolish woman can usually find friends with similar attitudes who will gladly reinforce her foolishness. Because she hates instruction, she falls into many bad habits and sins. She dresses carelessly, spends her money frivolously, and wrongs her own soul in the process. She likes to flaunt herself by wearing clothes that are too tight, too short, too low, too flamboyant, or just plain inappropriate. When a Christian woman wears something too revealing, it will be a sexual distraction for the men, exasperating to the other women, or both. But it is not displaying wisdom.

In stark contrast to the foolish woman is the wise woman. She fears the Lord, is not wise in her own eyes, departs from evil—even if it means departing from "the cool"; she is sensible, teachable, and loves her own soul. She cares more about what God thinks of her than men's opinions. She considers it a glory to be obedient to God, and she thinks pastorally about the world and about the state of her own soul. When she is choosing what to wear, she thinks about whether it would be "wise" to wear or not. How will it affect others? Is it appropriate for the occasion? Will it draw too much attention to her? Is it lovely?

While the foolish woman knows what men want (and she might even deliver it), the wise woman also knows how men think. She can see the difference between a wise man and a foolish one, and she is not in the market for a fool. She knows that if she pursues God with wisdom, He will bring her a wise man at the right time.

Wisdom dresses to be attractive, not seductive. She chooses clothing that is lovely, practical, and within her means. She doesn't buy a dress that will fit after she loses five pounds (and wear it in the meantime), but a dress that fits now. She is not suckered into impulsive purchases, but she thinks it over. She tries things on and checks in the dressing room to see how they look when she sits in them, when she bends over, when she walks. She chooses things that she knows will be adornments, not distractions. She looks chaste because she is chaste, and she loves virtue and sexual purity.

The church has always had to address the issue of modesty. It is nothing new. An old Puritan once said that "Some women dress as though they wanted the devil to fall in love with them." The foolish woman flatters and flirts; the naïve woman often makes foolish choices because of lack of wisdom. But the wise woman is blessed in the Lord. She has resolved to have nothing in her closet that would displease God, reflect poorly on her parents or her church, embarrass her wise friends, or make her look like a fool. That means she considers the importance of beauty, good taste, femininity, and refinement, as well as the issue of modesty.

Connected to modesty is the whole issue of sexual purity. The naive woman is shocked that anyone might view her in a sexual manner at all. The fool is provocative and knows it. But the wise woman understands that the way she dresses is an outworking of how she views and values her own purity. She is not interested in having multiple relationships with guys she does not respect. She is not interested in preserving her virginity "technically" while losing her own self-respect. She has a high view of the marriage bed and keeps herself pure both physically and mentally. She doesn't laugh at crass jokes or watch filthy movies. She doesn't dress like a woman looking for attention, and if some poor fellow tries to give her the wrong kind of attention, he won't get far.

Sexual purity extends to include books, magazines, music, and movies. It is inconsistent with masturbation and excludes porn, on the internet or otherwise. To dress with a Christian worldview, you must have a Christian worldview, and this affects everything we do.

And though we obviously think of sexual purity in terms of the opposite sex, it also is necessary to mention girlfriends. I have counseled enough young women who struggle with this that I should mention it here. Though healthy friendships are a positive good, a woman who is too emotionally dependent on other women is in a dangerous place. When women need a lot of physical contact from other women, whether it is back-rubbing, playing with each other's hair, or just being too huggy-kissy, it can be a red flag. At best, it is a sign of insecurity which will creep out the guys, concern the other girls, and make everyone uncomfortable. At worst, it is an early stage of what could become an unhealthy dependence that could lead to lesbianism. (But more on women's relationships in chapter 14.)

The way we dress sends a message to everyone about the kind of women we are. Learn the language, so you'll be sending the right signals.

CHAPTER 10

What Kind of Man Are You Looking For?

You might answer, "I'm not looking for a man!" But let's be honest about this. Of course you are looking for a man, and there is not one thing wrong with that. The wrong would be for you to flat out deny it. Now I don't think it is godly, healthy, or wise to be *obsessed* with watching for the right man to show up. But it is only natural for a woman who wants to be married to have her eyes open; a wise woman is paying attention. The important thing is to know *what kind of man* you are looking for and to keep from being tricked into thinking you have found him when you haven't.

Because of loneliness, women are tempted to respond to the wrong kind of man. And as I have said before, there is one thing worse than being unmarried (actually there are lots of things), and that is being married to the wrong man. I have talked with many miserable married women over the years. Why did they get married in the first place? Sometimes they saw him as a ticket out of their hard circumstances, but in reality he was a ticket to newer and harder circumstances. Marrying someone for the wrong reason will never lead to long-term happiness.

We have all heard funny descriptions of the ideal Christian man. One of my favorites is "tall, dark, rich, and reformed." Ah, you think, if only there were enough of that kind to go around! But the truth is, most women are not really that fussy. I have heard a woman complain about some of the Christian men in the community, but then when one of those same men showed an interest in her, she suddenly did not care about those things she had so freely criticized before. But though height or hair line may not be important, spiritual qualities are *not* to be overlooked for the sake of a relationship.

For starters, a Christian woman should marry a Christian man. That seems simple enough, but sometimes a woman can rationalize on this point. "Well, he goes to church sometimes." That is not enough to determine if he is a man of faith. "He was brought up Roman Catholic, but I'm not sure if he still is a practicing Catholic." A Protestant woman should not consider marrying a Catholic. "He is really nice, so I think he must be a Christian." That is certainly not enough evidence. "He was baptized as an infant, so he must be a Christian." Yes, but what kind of Christian? The kind who goes to hell? Marriage is much too important a connection to make with someone who has a different or nonexistent faith. Do not be swayed by a fun personality to overlook a man's spiritual condition. Besides, the Bible makes it clear that we are not to be unequally yoked.

So once you have determined that he is of the same faith, you have to consider what kind of Christian he is. Does he read his Bible? Does he do what it says? Is he a faithful church member? Does he tithe? Is he growing? Do you see him sharing his faith? Is he involved in the life of the congregation? Believe it or not, some men will play the part to get themselves a Christian wife, so you want to know that his faith is genuine. Not every man is called to be a leader in the church; but every husband is called to be a leader in his home. Can you see yourself being led by him?

The Bible requires wives to submit to their own husbands, so a woman ought to marry a man that she respects. If she respects him, she will be able to freely submit to him. If he is the kind of man who is eager to please and obey God, she should not have trouble following him. The Bible also requires wives to respect and honor their husbands. So it follows that a woman should marry a man that she can easily look up to. Respect and honor are far more easily rendered to a respectable, honorable man. This is something a woman should know about a man before she allows herself to fall in love with him. If she is emotionally attached, she is in real danger of rationalizing these things away. But once she is married to him, there will be no excuses for disrespect.

Because of the wonderful way God made the world, what one woman respects in a man, another may not. In other words, some women can be led by men who in no way could lead someone else. A woman with a strong personality will need a man with a lot of horsepower to lead her. She doesn't want to marry a man whom she will always have to be leading herself. Though she may not mind at first, it will get old very fast. If she is a hard charger, she needs to marry someone who is more of one. A woman is called to follow, support, and help her husband, and that is difficult to do if a wife is miles ahead hollering, "Come on, you can catch up!" This applies to strength of personality, spiritual zeal, intellectual gifts, and initiative. Though a man may wish his wife had more of these things so she could keep up with him, it is far worse to have a wife who is way ahead of her husband.

Online dating services have questionnaires that deal with all kinds of aspects of personality and gifts. Though much of this is valuable, we have to be careful not to view the way a man and woman come together as some sort of formula. Obviously they should share similar tastes, likes, and dislikes when it comes to cultural preferences. But complementing someone is not necessarily the same as being identical in every way. A woman should know which things are nonnegotiable and which things are indifferent to her. For example, if she is not a camper, but she wouldn't mind becoming a camper, then that falls in the indifferent category. But if she must live by the ocean, and he is planning to live in the Midwest, then that is nonnegotiable. But sometimes a woman thinks he is so wonderful that she will gladly give up living by the ocean. What was nonnegotiable becomes indifferent. These things will vary from person to person, and a woman should have these things sorted out in her mind before she agrees to get married.

Other important things should be considered. How does he treat his mother? How does he treat his other family members? How does he handle money? Is he a hard worker? Is he self-disciplined? Does he live for others? Does he have a temper? What about personal habits? Is he a slob? What about his sexual history? Does he look at pornography? Does he have high (meaning *godly*) standards for entertainment?

Especially in the cases of using online dating services, many women don't really know the answers to many of these questions before they get married. And obviously, once they are married, it is too late. This can be particularly true in cross-cultural marriages. A woman needs to understand all the cultural expectations her husband will bring into the marriage. What is his view of childrearing and the role of women in the home? What about family celebrations? Is he planning for his parents to live with them? These things might not come up in a couple months of email exchanges, so be thorough and be wise. Though a cross-cultural marriage to a fellow believer is entirely lawful, it will have unique challenges, so be careful. Even a culture that speaks the same language as yours can be entirely different. If a woman from the South marries a man from New England, she may be surprised to find out what deep differences exist even within our own country. How much more if he is from an entirely different country. This is not said to discourage cross-cultural marriages, but simply to encourage women to do their homework before they fall in love.

Finally, a woman should marry a man she finds attractive. That does not mean that she thinks he would be voted the world's sexiest man and put on the cover of some magazine. But *she* should find him attractive. She does not have to think he is the most handsome man in the church. But she should not marry him unless she thinks he is, as Solomon put it in the Song of Songs, an apple tree in the forest. He should be all she wants. On the other hand, if he repulses her physically, then no matter how godly he is, it is an unwise match. She might find him unattractive at first, but if she gets to know him and then finds him appealing, she could go ahead. However, it is a mistake to think that these things don't matter, and that somehow it is more spiritual to just ignore the physical. God did not make us that way. Chemistry isn't everything, but it is still important. A woman has to keep this all in perspective: is he a godly man she can follow and is she attracted to him?

As a woman navigates this, she must remember that in all of life we are to walk by faith. God has promised to never leave us or forsake us. If there is no man on the horizon right now, or the ones who "fit the bill" don't seem to be interested, it is important to remember that God is overseeing it all. Trust Him and do not lower the standard because of loneliness. You will find it is much too high a price to pay.

CHAPTER 11

Keep Your Heart

We've all known women who have gotten hurt in relationships that didn't work out. Looking back, it's easy to wonder what went wrong. How did she let herself get too emotionally involved before there was any kind of serious commitment? I've seen women get hurt even when the men had never given them the least bit of encouragement. Obviously, in such a case, a woman had let herself develop a serious "crush" on someone who had not shown any interest in her. Keeping your heart requires watching your thought life and not daydreaming about what *might* happen. But it also requires some basic teaching on men and women.

One of the central ways for a woman to guard her heart and keep from getting hurt in relationships or nonrelationships is to understand the differences between men and women. God has created us with design features that are different, and yet complement us. Getting a grasp on some of these things won't ensure that you will never get hurt, but it will help you exercise wisdom in understanding the men you deal with.

First of all, men have a different view of the relationship than women do. Wives are called by God to be helpers to their husbands. Because of the creation mandate given to men and women, God has uniquely equipped each of us to do what He has called us to do. Women are designed to work well in their support role, cheering their men on to do great things, being intuitive about what he needs, thinking practically about what will keep the boat afloat, and being detail-oriented. This is why women make good wives and mothers. I'm certainly not saying that women can't do anything else; but because of the way women can think intuitively and practically, and because of their capacity to multitask, women can run households (and a lot of other things) in a way that (generally speaking) men can't.

Men are generally analytical, not intuitive, theoretical rather than practical. They have a one-track mind, and they usually get lost in a conversation with a woman when she jumps from one topic to another without providing the necessary antecedent. Men think in terms of accomplishing a mission, and when that is done, they move on to the next one.

So how does all this connect to the view of a relationship? For a woman, the relationship to the man is central. He *is* her mission. She is called to help him in whatever it is he is doing. During a courtship, the man views the relationship as the mission. But once the courtship-mission is accomplished, and the girl is won, he then is able to get back to his work, whatever his calling is, and enjoy her help. She brings delight to his life. But when he gets back to work, she continues to focus on the relationship, on *him*, because he *is* her job and calling. He must focus on his mission. It is important to see the difference in our God-designed callings here. Women can become defensive and unhappy about this if they misunderstand it. It does not mean that a woman loves a man more than he loves her. It is not about that at all. It is about calling and mission assignment. This is simply the way God made us.

This difference in perspective can easily be seen in novels or movies written by and for men compared to novels or movies written for women (commonly called the chick flick). A movie for men is about the mission, the adventure, the war, the gold, or the spy ring. Though it may have a relationship in it, the relationship is not the main thing. In a film for women, the relationship *is* the plot. It is all about them getting together, and if there is a mission or adventure, that is a side plot. Whether it is a cheesy grocery store romance novel or great literature like *Pride and Prejudice,* women like the story about the relationship itself. That's where the action is.

Men and women's sexual wiring is also different. Men are built to be initiators, and women are designed to be responders. As George Gilder helpfully points out in his book, *Men and Marriage,*[1] women are wired for a long-term sexual relationship that extends from the time they begin their menstrual cycle, through marriage, pregnancy, childbirth, breastfeeding, childrearing, to the time the children leave home. Men, on the other hand, have a short-term sexual cycle that lasts about as long as the sexual act itself. That explains why the man without sense in Proverbs is drawn to the harlot. He is certainly not thinking about how he will put the kid through college; he is thinking about a very short-term good time. Of course, God has called the man to settle down with one woman and submit his short-term cycle to her long-term cycle, sticking with her through the pregnancy, childbirth, childrearing, and the college tuition payments. That is the glory of God's design.

Men are seduced physically, attracted by sight, while women are seduced emotionally, attracted by tenderness and thoughtful attention. Thus we have scriptural warnings to the men to avoid the strange woman, the evil woman, the whorish woman. And we have scriptural warnings to women to dress modestly and to be chaste. An immodest woman is disregarding the Word, and she doesn't love the brothers. A man who is

1. George Gilder, *Men and Marriage* (Gretna: Pelican Publishing, 1986), 8–9.

chasing after the adulteress is also disregarding the Word, and he is destroying the community. Both are wicked and destructive in their own way.

The woman's primary need in a relationship is security and love. In the same way, a man has a deep need for respect and admiration. Of course, men need love and women need respect, but not in the same way. This is why women are more interested (usually) than men are in communication. Women want to be understood; they want to be listened to. This gives them a feeling of love and security in the relationship. A woman wants someone who will provide for her and protect her. Men are hungry for their wives to praise them, to appreciate them for their accomplishments and abilities. They are built to need respect. While women are more aware of their emotions, men are more aware of their appetites.

So how does all this relate to keeping your heart? It explains how unmarried men and women view the need for marriage differently. An unmarried woman wants someone she can follow and help; an unmarried man wants someone to provide for and protect. A man may pursue a relationship as a mission, employing all the methods that will appeal to the woman. But he is not by nature usually romantic, emotional, and feeling-oriented. Friendships with men are far more sexually charged than most women realize. Just because you are friends does not mean you are neuter.

Because of a woman's need to be a communicator, she can confide too much in a man before she is protected by a marriage covenant. She may be manipulated by him into this, or she may rush ahead herself. Because a woman is intuitive and compassionate, she can feel sorry for someone who confides in her, and this can lead her to get into an unwise relationship. Many women have fallen in love with men for whom they have no respect at all. At the same time, a man who is a manipulator may know exactly what he is doing and get a woman to give him what he wants without the protection of a marriage covenant.

Because of the single woman's hunger for companionship, and because she wants to be needed, she can rush in to "help a brother" in ways that are inappropriate, making him meals, doing his laundry, cleaning his apartment, ironing his shirts. She may think that she is making him want her, but he may think that he has a pretty good deal in a free housekeeper.

Women have a deep attraction to male leadership, and that is why they can respond to men who may be leading in the wrong direction. At least they are going somewhere! So a woman must guard herself from simply being attracted to the raw masculinity of leadership without paying close attention to where he is going. Many men lead women into sin and disobedience. Think of all the women you know who have fallen away from the faith because of a man with "leadership skills." Being a leader is not enough. Is he leading you to Christ or away from Him? This attraction to leadership is the only explanation for the number of women who become attached to dictatorial or disobedient men. Why do so many unmarried women continue to stay with men who mistreat them? "But I love him," is the common answer. Sad to say, many single women who have grown up with dictatorial fathers marry the same kind of man, and thus perpetuate the problem.

Keeping your heart means not giving your heart away too readily, not being an easy audience, not being too easily impressed, and not being too readily available for attention from the wrong sort of man. Christian women should render respect to men who are respectable, not men that they hope will become respectable. Remember, wives are commanded to submit to their *own* husbands. The command is not to women generally to submit to men generally. The Christian faith protects women in this way like no other religion or system on earth. Though it is caricatured as a faith that mistreats women, it is quite the reverse, bestowing honor on the woman and providing for her protection from men in general.

While men need to guard against the woman who flatters, women need to guard against the man who is thoughtful and kind. This may sound funny at first, but a woman can be drawn into a relationship because "he is so nice." Maybe he fixes her flat tire or helps her unload her groceries, but the next thing you know, she has become attached to him emotionally. She might not even know whether he is a Christian or not. Women need to guard and keep their hearts so they can determine if this really is a godly man or just a nice guy who knows how to play his cards. This may be a male version of flattery and flirtation. If a woman is hungry for it, she may easily fall for a man for all the wrong reasons. But a relationship that is honoring to God won't be built on a foundation of flattery or flirtation.

Of course, there is always risk involved in any relationship. But a woman ought to feel pretty sure about what she is doing before she lets her heart get entangled. It's much easier to dive in than it is to climb out.

CHAPTER 12

Are You Desirable?

If you want God to provide you with a husband, you have to consider whether you are the kind of woman that the kind of man you want to marry would want to marry. Shall I go over that again? What kind of woman is that kind of man looking for? Are you that kind of woman? Are you desirable? This is a delicate topic in our egalitarian age, and so I approach it gingerly.

In a previous chapter I addressed the need for single women to be productive and fruitful members of the church community. So I won't go into that again here. Suffice it to say that if you want to marry a *godly* man, he will be looking for a *godly* woman. So that is the first and most important thing. You should be cultivating a healthy Christian life.

But there are other issues. What else is a godly man looking for? He will be looking for an attractive woman. Are you attractive? Some women have false illusions about how attractive they are, and so they set their sights on the most attractive men in the community. You should be realistic about your attractiveness as well as your potential. If you are a moderately attractive woman, you should assume that you will marry a moderately attractive man. If you are a knockout, then it's fine to assume you will marry someone equally remarkable. But don't kid yourself.

Some mythology floating around goes like this: a godly man doesn't care about the externals. He just looks on the heart. So if I am godly, it doesn't matter whether I am pretty or not. But that is a myth. The Bible describes some women as *beautiful*; for example, Sarah, Rebekah, Rachel, and Abigail are each called beautiful. It is not unspiritual or less spiritual to care about beauty. It is sinful to become vain or idolatrous about it, but the Christian worldview embraces the ideas of truth, goodness, and beauty. We can't just appreciate the truth and goodness part and dismiss beauty. That is rebelling against the way God designed the world. So a Christian woman should be careful to be orthodox (that's the truth part) and good (that's the moral part), and she should also be beautiful (that's the part I'm talking about in this chapter).

Some women think their looks are unrelated to the fact that they are still unmarried. Or they think they are as attractive as they can possibly be. But the truth is they could do a lot to improve their looks. If you sit in a mall and just watch the people go by, you will see that the average American woman today is overweight, unfeminine, and slobby. Christian women should repudiate such a lifestyle and embrace the feminine and the beautiful.

Consider what you could do to be more beautiful. This is not ungodly or worldly wisdom. This is simply the way God made the world. We are creatures. We love the true, the good, and the beautiful. So what could you do to be more attractive? Do you need to lose a few (or more) pounds? Or do you need to quit fussing about your weight and stop working out so much? What if you got your hair cut in a cuter, more up-to-date style? Could you dress in a more flattering manner? Do you need to get your teeth straightened? Let's face it: men are attracted to beautiful women.

Many Christian women are overlooking this, telling themselves that it is more spiritual to think beauty is irrelevant, but that is not true. Some Christian women are smothering their beauty, hiding it, or keeping it camouflaged for various reasons. It is hiding under thirty extra pounds, or it is simply hidden behind an unkempt appearance. Consider getting an objective opinion about this. Maybe there are some simple things you could do that would improve your appearance. I'm certainly not advocating cosmetic surgery, unless it is for something that is truly a handicap and cannot be fixed without extreme measures. But things like braces, facial hair removal, teeth whitening, removing scars or warts, getting some new clothes, or losing some weight are all lawful and helpful. (Getting breast implants is in another category all together; I am not advocating such things—unless of course it is fixing a serious problem, like reconstructive surgery after breast cancer treatments.)

So, do an honest evaluation of your appearance. It's amazing what a little makeup can do. If you are prone to dress in a style called the thrift-store look, press on to something less dated. Do you dress like your great aunt who was a school marm? Branch out a little. Update your wardrobe. Have your hair styled. Wear some perfume. There is absolutely no reason for Christian women to be dumpy. And unless you are one in a thousand, you probably need a little makeup and a hair style to look as beautiful as you can. To deny the fact that men appreciate beautiful women is to argue with gravity. If you are plain, you can still use all in your power to bring out your best. If you have a lot of natural beauty, be a good steward of it. This is common sense.

Of course it is possible to overachieve in this area. A woman who is overdone can be overwhelming to everyone. I am not advocating wearing so much perfume to the party that it arrives five minutes before you do. Easy does it. I'm simply encouraging women to take their responsibility to be attractive seriously. Don't put it off. Get to work.

But in saying all these things, I want to carefully qualify it this way: if you just don't like makeup or perfume, I am not suggesting that you must. Perhaps, in the providence of God, you will marry someone who doesn't like them either. I'm simply suggesting that you come out of the woodwork. If you are chubby, then you will probably marry someone who is chubby too. I am not suggesting that everyone has to be thin, but women need to be realistic about how their appearance relates to the desire for marriage. In this age, when women can lurch into eating disorders, I am wary of urging any kind of weight loss project without a few warnings. Get an objective opinion. Ask your mom. Be smart about this. Eating disorders are the result of insecurity and self-absorption. Be wise here.

Another consideration is personality. If you are a quiet person who sits on the sidelines, chances are good that the handsome man with the gregarious personality will never notice you. Just as the handsome men will be drawn to the beautiful women, the outgoing men will be drawn to the vivacious women with lots of personality. So drag yourself out of the corner and be a little more interesting. If you don't have anything to talk about, start reading so that you will. Prepare ahead of time so you'll have a few possible topics in hand before you go to the party. It's great to be a good listener; but you have to be a participant as well. If you are shy and unwilling to change, accept the fact that you will probably not end up with an outgoing extrovert. These are natural consequences of our gifts and traits.

Then there is the question of domesticity. Would you be able to run a household if you were given the opportunity? Do you know how to cook? shop? iron? set a table? clean a bathroom? work with a budget? Can you handle the responsibility of managing a home? Do you know anything about children? decorating? hospitality? These are important questions. If you want to be a wife and mother, you should be honing your homemaking skills now, preparing for the day when you will be the mistress of a home. The domestic arts are vital to making a house into a real home, a place that is a refuge and oasis in a hectic world. If you are not domestic at all, why do you think you would make a good helper? Get to work on this and put domesticity on your agenda.

I say all these things to promote hard-headed thinking and realistic self-evaluation, not to bring discouragement or cause morbid introspection. Get serious about becoming the kind of woman who will attract the kind of man you want.

Someone may tell you to just wear tighter, shorter skirts to attract a man. That might work. But it's not going to attract the kind of man you want to marry. On the other hand, if people are giving you this sort of advice because you're wearing prairie-muffin dresses, it may not be such bad advice after all, unless you want to marry a prairie-muffin kind of guy. In that case, keep the calico and don't worry about any of this.

CHAPTER 13

Loving the Brothers

In Titus 2, Paul exhorts Titus to "speak the things which are proper for sound doctrine." In his list of instructions, Paul specifies that the old men are to be "sober, reverent, temperate, sound in faith, in love, in patience" (v. 2), and the young men are to be sober-minded—sensible (v. 6). Now it seems to me that as we consider how the women are to treat the men in the church, we should take Paul's instructions into account. In other words, the sisters should be promoting "sober-mindedness" among the brothers, whether young or old. By this I do not mean that the sisters are to be teaching the young men. No. Rather, I mean that their behavior toward the brothers should not be counterproductive to Paul's instructions.

Just a few verses later, Paul exhorts all believers to deny ungodliness and to live "soberly, righteously, and godly." So the behavior of the single women toward the single men should be characterized by a careful attentiveness to God's Word, showing all reverence. Let me break this down into a few specific areas.

First, women should dress in a manner that promotes chastity and displays a godly discretion and modesty. A modestly dressed woman is not a distraction to the brothers. There is a difference between being attractive and dressing to attract. Christian women should *adorn* (or beautify) themselves modestly with propriety and moderation (1 Tim. 2:9). This implies self-discipline, self-control, and wisdom. A seductress beautifies herself also, but she "lies in wait as for a victim" (Prov. 23:28). A Christian woman should not be easily confused with a hooker, but the way some women dress today, it is sometimes hard to tell.

Let me be specific here. Our culture does not promote nor does it approve of chastity. Adultery and fornication are the norm, and one walk through a department store tells you that the clothing designers are doing their best to promote ungodliness. Just today, my daughter and I saw a T-shirt that had the words "pinch me" written across the chest. It's not even subtle or suggestive anymore, but crass and impudent. Though most Christian women would not be tempted to wear that T-shirt, there is still far too much immodesty in our ranks. When a Christian woman (married or single) wears something too short or too tight, or she is bending over and giving everyone in a five-mile radius the view down her shirt, it will either be a sexual distraction for the young men, an annoyance to the other women, or both. But it is not displaying wisdom.

Second, when women are flirtatious, it is not treating the brothers with wisdom. A flirt is a flatterer, bestowing too much attention on the men in a provocative way. The film industry has been diligent to teach women how to flirt in different settings: here's how you flirt in a bar, here's how you flirt at work, etc. Christian women can easily modify the techniques for how to flirt with a Christian brother.

A simple standard is this: treat all the brothers like you would if you were married or if they were married. In other words, you don't want to treat a brother in a way that would be entirely unacceptable if you or he were married. He is someone's future husband, right? So you don't want to be embarrassed by your own behavior down the road.

But what about *friendships* with men? Certainly it is healthy for Christians to have friendships with both men and women. But consider that it is hazardous to have one-on-one friendships with men because more often than not, one of you will start viewing the other as something more than a friend. If it happens to both at the same time, then it can blossom into a courtship. But if it only happens to one of you, that means the other person will get hurt. Cultivate friendships in groups. Once you start pairing off, you are in danger of becoming too attached. If it is a mutual attachment, you can be thankful that you've survived a potentially dangerous situation. Unfortunately, that doesn't always happen. So don't grow fond in an unprotected setting. I have no idea how many times I have talked with women who were crushed when they found out that their "close friend" became engaged to someone else. Guard your heart and keep a friendly distance.

Women are built to respond, not to initiate; to be sought after, not to be the ones doing the chasing. Though women may think it's up to them to make this relationship happen, that is a bad precedent in a marriage. If you are really the one who has to get this thing off the ground, then you'll probably have to be the one to lead in many other ways once you are married. Husbands are to lead their wives, so beware of a relationship in which you are the leader. This is a very bad start.

Be careful of your relationships to married men as well. Don't look to them as your spiritual head. Don't single them out regularly for advice or help. Rather, cultivate friendships with couples, families, and with individual women.

Years ago I was meeting once a week with an unmarried woman, helping her get established in her Christian faith. We met on an evening when my husband had a regular commitment, so she seldom saw him when she came over. One night he arrived while she was still there, and she said to him, "I feel really close to Nancy, but I don't feel close to you at all." My husband smiled and said, "Good. You're not supposed to!" This, as you can imagine, came as a surprise to her, but after we explained it to her, she saw our point. I don't want my husband having friendships with women, and he doesn't want me having friendships with men. But as a couple, we are friends with many men and women together. This is one way we protect our marriage.

Unmarried women appreciate the input from and fellowship with men, and they should. So seek out friendships with families, not just with other unmarried men and women. You can get to know them as a couple. Keep your distance. Don't become dependent on any man who is not your father or your husband. Learn to love the brothers in a way that will be a blessing to everyone.

CHAPTER 14

Loving the Competition

While listening to an audio series, I was struck by an offhand comment made by the speaker: she said that women are some of the worst misogynists in the world. This is a stark reality. Just consider the women's movement, which is fueled by a woman-hating agenda. It has had a generation in which to work its magic, and it has failed in a spectacular way. Not only has it failed to create unity among women, but it has rather divided and alienated them.

Unfortunately, this woman-hating attitude is not limited to secular society. It can and does exist among Christian sisters, where criticism, envy, and distrust can destroy the possibility of Christian fellowship. Though there may be a surface congeniality, a deep love of the sisters is frequently nonexistent. Where there should be kindness and love, there is instead "contentions, jealousies, outbursts of wrath, selfish ambitions, backbitings, whisperings, conceits, tumults" (2 Cor. 12:20). Women tend to be far more critical of the other women than they are of men. But, by the grace of God, Christian women have the opportunity to build a climate of friendship, encouragement, and support among the sisters in the church community. What is it that causes women to be so quick to be critical, envious, and distrustful of one another?

I believe part of the answer has to do with a sinful sense of competition among sisters that keeps them from fulfilling their obligation to love one another. This competition centers, of course, around men. The single women compete for attention from the single men, and the married women can carry on the competition in other forms. When sisters are viewed as the competition, no wonder there is a bent toward criticism and envy.

Woman was created for man, and since the fall, man has had a roving eye. The young women jostle for attention from the young men and begin to view their sisters who get the attention as self-centered, immodest, flirtatious, etc. And by the time they're in their thirties or even in their twenties, the pattern is set. The problem here is theological. If God is truly sovereign, as we believe He is, then He has ordained who will marry whom and when. In other words, the sisters are not competition in any way whatsoever. Though you can sin as though you are competing, you really are not in a competition for a husband. This means that the Christian woman can overcome the tendency toward competition and have a sincere love for the sisters.

The flirt is someone who tries to gain the attention of men in whom she has no serious interest, just so she can see that "all systems are working." She may be able to gather a group of men around her with little effort; meanwhile, the other sisters look on with positive annoyance. They may try to legitimize their annoyance by pointing out her real or imagined sins, but this necessarily requires attributing motives, and leads to gossip, backbiting, envying, whisperings, or real strife. Sometimes the woman with the group of men around her is really not flirting, but she's just very attractive and engaging. In this case, she may need to be more actively discouraging to the young men. But in the meanwhile, the sisters should not get ticked off at her.

This envy can be fueled at all kinds of community events, particularly at weddings and showers. But the single women should not stay away from such events because they can't handle seeing everyone else getting married and having children. If they confine themselves to the fringes, they'll not overcome this temptation.

Women tend to confide too much in one another. Call it over-sharing. They shouldn't be surprised when some of their confidences get shared elsewhere. Be careful about talking too much about the men you are interested in, about past relationships, or about your own personal struggles. Share with people who can help, but don't just vent. If you talk about the man you're interested in, and find out that someone else likes him too, this can obviously lead to competition, envy, hurt feelings, and all the rest. It's wiser to keep it to yourself. If you need input, talk to a very trusted friend, maybe your mom or the pastor's wife. Don't talk about the guys with the girls. Sometimes this seems like innocent entertainment, but if one of the girls ends up marrying one of the guys you said was a dweeb, you'll be sorry you said anything about it.

Another thing that can cause disruption of fellowship is when one woman gets married and becomes very patronizing to the unmarried women. Her old friends, rather than wishing her well, would prefer to kick her in the ankle. This is like Lydia in *Pride and Prejudice* when she offers to find husbands for her older sisters.

Obviously, God did not design us to be envious and distrustful of one another. Women should reject the temptation to view the other women as competition. If you find that you can't really rejoice when a friend gets engaged, then you've probably got a case of envy. Even if you were not competing for the same man, if you are critical of her, of her choice of husband, or of the wedding details, these are signs that you are being envious. Confess it! Her story is not your story, and God is writing both. Be the kind of character that you admire, not one of those petty characters that annoy every reader.

Sad to say, women who are competitive and envious before marriage will carry the tendency straight over into marriage and continue to compete, whether it is over having the best kids, the best house, or the best figure. This is a sign of insecurity and neediness. How much better it would be to deal with such things before you are married.

Instead of being misogynists, Christian women have the best reason to love the sisters: we are all in Christ.

> Therefore, as the elect of God, holy and beloved, put on tender mercies, kindness, humility, meekness, longsuffering; . . . But above all these things put on love, which is the bond of perfection. (Col. 3:12, 14)

> Let us not become conceited, provoking one another, envying one another. (Gal. 5:26)

CHAPTER 15

Setting Standards of Personal Holiness

If you have grown up in a godly Christian home, then your parents taught you and instilled in you a set of godly standards for Christian living. If you really understood why they were protecting you, and if you internalized those standards, then you have been blessed.

On the other hand, if you grew up in a home where your parents wanted you to figure things out for yourself, you probably have a different story. But in either case, a single woman needs to have a clear-cut set of standards for herself. These governing principles will help keep her life simple.

Some women have to learn all these things the hard way, like the kid who burns his finger on the hot stove. It's better not to get burned, but now you know.

Standards are not automatic, and some women have high standards for themselves, but they don't know how to enforce them when it comes to living in community. So here are a few things to think about.

Titus 2:11–12 helps us get started. "For the grace of God that brings salvation has appeared to all men, teaching us that, denying ungodliness and worldly lusts, we should live soberly, righteously, and godly in the present age." I like the way the NIV renders verse 12: "It teaches us to say 'No' to ungodliness and worldly passions, and to live self-controlled, upright and godly lives in this present age." Christian women need to learn to say "no" to many things, and it is the grace of God that teaches us this important detail. Having standards of personal holiness is going to involve saying "no" a lot, mostly to ourselves!

Women can be easily deceived, particularly by men, and they have a particular phobia about hurting feelings. Let's say someone calls and invites you to go out to dinner and to a movie. You don't want to go, but you don't want to hurt the poor guy's feelings, so you say "yes." Or you say you're busy (which is not technically true), and then he calls back in a few days to try again. Sooner or later you either have to go out with him, or you have to say "no." "No, thanks" will work too. But you may not lie.

Hurting the poor guy's feelings is a myth that somehow is perpetuated among women from one generation to the next. But the truth is, though he may be disappointed, chances are good he will get over it pretty quickly and ask someone else. I doubt you have destroyed his male ego in one fell swoop. But how do you say no? Here's a real life practice scenario for you.

"Hi."

"Hi."

"Would you like to go to the rodeo with me Friday night?"

"No, thanks."

"Why? Don't you like rodeos?"

"Actually, it's not really about the rodeo. I appreciate you as a friend, but I'm not interested in being in a dating relationship with you."

"Oh. Thanks for telling me."

"No problem."

Now that wasn't so painful. Actually, it was painful, but once it's over, it doesn't seem so painful anymore. Practice this! Then you won't end up out for the evening with someone you have no interest in.

What about the persistent guy?

"Hi."

"Hi."

"Want to come to my apartment for dinner and see the pictures of my trip?"

"No, thanks."

"Ah, come on. It will be great. My pictures are fantastic."

"No doubt they are. But I'd rather not."

"Are you sure?"

"Yes, I'm sure."

"Would you reconsider?"

"No, I wouldn't."

"But why don't you want to come watch my slides."

"I think I said no thanks."

Now some of you are going to think, "Oh, but that is so rude!" Yes, that was very rude. He was completely out of line to be so persistent. He should have just accepted the first "No thanks" and pressed on. "But," you'll say, "I wasn't talking about him. *She* was so rude!"

There you go, just as I said. You've just proven my point! Women don't recognize where the rudeness really lies. When a man exerts pressure on a woman, that is a signal to speak directly. And you should not feel bad about doing so. If you want to feel bad, then feel bad about all the times that you should have said no and were too wimpy to do it.

But how do you determine which ones to say no to and which ones to say yes to? First off, you should not date unbelievers. Period. Don't tell yourself that it's dating evangelism. That's a proven formula for failure and regret. (Okay, some of you are going to think of a case where there was a real conversion. I'm not denying that happens. But we all know that more often than conversion, there is compromise and sin.) If you know someone who is interested in finding out more about the faith, hand him off to a brother as fast as you can. If you don't know for sure what kind of Christian he is, don't agree to a big date. Suggest meeting for coffee instead. Then you can come and go independently, and you haven't committed to a whole evening with someone you're not sure about.

Maybe you will decide, as I did, that I wasn't going to date anyone unless it was someone I thought I might marry. That made my life very simple and uncomplicated.

But standards include more than *who* you'll go out with. *Where* will you go? Where will you *not* go? How late will you stay out? What kind of parties will you attend? Having standards helps you figure these things out.

"Would you like to go out Friday night?"
"Maybe. Where?"
"Oh, I don't know. Maybe a movie?"
"Which movie?"
"How 'bout *Mary Poppins*?"
"Okay. Where will we be watching it?"
"My apartment."
"Will your roommates be there?"
"No. They're gone for the weekend."
"Ah. No thanks."

Don't be afraid to ask questions. Find out. Say no. It is your conscience that you must keep clean. If you watch a filthy movie because you were too embarrassed to say anything and too timid to leave, then your own conscience is guilty. You can't blame it on the host. You're not a little kid. You need to have standards and a backbone to enforce them.

Here are a few suggestions: Don't entertain men in your house if you're alone. Have group activities. Don't go to men's apartments unless it is a group event. And even if it's a group event, leave at a decent hour. If you stay too late, you might get too comfortable. Don't laugh at dirty jokes. Insist on a high tone. Don't get stuck at parties that have a low moral tone. Look around and ask yourself, "Are these my people?" If not, leave. Have a curfew for yourself. Don't be afraid to stand up for yourself.

My father-in-law uses this illustration to make the point: Sin is like a cliff that we can fall off. Forgiveness is like an ambulance at the bottom. If we sin, God will always forgive us. But it makes more sense to have a fence at the top of the cliff to keep us from falling. That fence is made up of our standards. Some Christians like to sit on the edge of the cliff and dangle their feet. They flirt with disaster and sometimes they fall. And though the ambulance is there to pick them up, they still get battered and hurt by the sin. So build a fence and stay away from the edge.

We are to be self-controlled people who take heed to our own souls. God has given us power over our own spirits. You do not have to give way to foolish behavior. But once you have given into it, it may be very difficult to get out. You may have made a habit of drinking too much, of watching cruddy movies, of getting physically involved with men who are not your husband or even your husband-to-be. This means you've fallen off the cliff. Don't stay down there. Get up. Get forgiveness. Then start building fences while you mend.

CHAPTER 16

Culture Building
and the Single Woman

One of my favorite Scriptures describing the place of women in a Christian culture is Psalm 144, verse 12b: "that our daughters may be as corner stones, polished after the similitude of a palace" (AV).

This is a lovely description of women who are living under the blessing of God. It is a considerable mercy for a culture to be able to boast of women like this, and a joy to be such a woman. This psalm ends by saying in verse 15, "Happy are the people who are in such a state; happy are the people whose God is the LORD!" Women like this are rare, but in a godly Christian culture, they should not be so rare. A culture with women like this has good reason to be happy.

All women, whether married or unmarried, are daughters. This means that the Scriptures speak to all of us. Single women can glean from this passage, just as they can from all of Scripture, but they can especially benefit from seeing themselves as daughters rather than as "singles." All that this passage implies is true for the unmarried, old or young. We should all take this to heart and strive to be the kind of women who can be described as polished cornerstones. So consider what this passage has to say to women in general.

As we all know, the cornerstone of a building is significant and impressive. It certainly is not one of the random stones in the wall. It is notable, recognized as not only an essential part, but also the most important part of the foundation. The Bible teaches that women have great significance in the Church, for good or for ill. The way they live before God will have a big impact on the Church. They can be used to bring great blessing, like the holy women described in 1 Peter 3:5 who "trusted in God"; or they can be silly women, like those in 2 Timothy 3:7 who are always learning but "never able to come to the knowledge of the truth." These are certainly not cornerstones. Neither are the women described in 1 Timothy 5:13–14 who, by being idle busybodies, give the adversary occasion to speak reproachfully. A marble cornerstone is far from silly. It has strength and stature, gravity and dignity.

Christian women, whether married or unmarried, necessarily have much to contribute to the establishment of a Christian culture. This occurs first and foremost in their homes, as they manage the little Christian culture for which they are responsible. This is, after all, where culture begins. We must not have a low view of what it takes to be a godly wife and mother. But even if a woman is living alone, unmarried and with no children, she is to manage her affairs in a decidedly Christian manner. This includes all the details. The idea is to let our theology affect our lives, inside and out. If all you have is a bedroom, take a look at it. What are you saying about your theology? Is it true? Or are you telling lies about God in your slovenliness? Having a Christian worldview in our head is not enough. We must live out all that we believe by the manner in which we conduct ourselves in all the little mundane things. Your house or apartment or bedroom is a picture of what you want to export and spread around to create a Christian culture.

Is it a good picture or a poor picture? If it is a poor picture, then it is time to remedy the situation. We are not to assume that in twenty years we will do something important culturally. We must begin now in our own bedrooms and kitchens and dining rooms and realize the significance of all our actions. We must take our duties seriously and go about our business with a sense of the importance of everything we are doing.

A daughter who is a polished cornerstone is no dummy. She loves truth and virtue, and she is a diligent student and Bible reader. She applies herself to intellectual pursuits and knows that learning to be domestic *includes* studying literature and history and math and science as well as learning the domestic arts. She loves the idea of home and embraces all that it encompasses. A single woman who has finished her formal education should not assume she is done with learning. She should press on to learn all she can about God and the world He has made. This should be a life-long pursuit of understanding truth, goodness, and beauty.

But what does it mean to be "polished after the similitude of a palace"? This implies refinement, beauty, and nobility. In other words, this isn't just a cornerstone in an unimportant building. It is the significant part of a very beautiful and central building; it's a palace, the seat of royalty. Refinement, or polish, has to do with the externalization of internal beauty, which includes appearance, manners, and conduct. This kind of woman is a lady. For example, she does not run with the men or after them. She knows that to chase men is to reverse God's designed order and to bring dishonor on herself. One wise father has said that if a woman gets the man she chases, she gets a fool. A polished, godly woman understands how to conduct herself with propriety, modesty, and confidence. This means she embraces much that our postmodern culture has pitched overboard. She may be an old-fashioned woman in that sense, but she is not backward or stuck in the nineteenth century when it comes to understanding the importance of Christian culture and how it relates to God's promises.

A woman who is polished has good taste. This is not the same thing as morality, but it is the direct consequence of morality. If you consider the abominable way women dress today, you can easily trace it as the direct result of our immoral culture. Women who want to be like polished marble must first apply themselves to virtue, but then they must study good manners. Manners have been described as love in the little things. Manners include how we dress, the way we walk, sit, eat, and converse with people. Christian courtesy applies in every situation. Good taste includes choices we make about aesthetics: our clothing, our surroundings, the books we read, the music we listen to, and so forth. Though not all people who have good taste are virtuous, virtuous people will mature in their good taste.

Loving beauty does not mean limiting it to the externals. Polished marble is beautiful, because it has gone through a beautifying process. For a Christian woman, this kind of beauty is in the inside first. External beauty is nothing if it is not connected to an internal beauty that comes from a gentle and quiet spirit. Do not suppose money can buy this. This internal beautification results in a radiant exterior. Christian women should want to be beautiful because this is God's gift. It is not self-centered and self-satisfying, but God-glorifying. A gentle and quiet spirit is an ornament that impresses God. It is a deferring beauty, not a grasping beauty.

Finally, this image suggests nobility because this is a marble cornerstone in a palace. This is what Israel wants for its daughters. Of course, we cannot alter the family we are in so that we can live in palaces. That is not what is suggested here. But we can be noble by having greatness of character. This kind of character is humble and obedient before God. A woman who conducts herself with this kind of stateliness would be comfortable in a palace. After all, our heavenly Father is king of the universe. We can live as though we really believe this. We can bring honor and glory to His name by the way we embrace His truth, His goodness, and His beauty. We can adorn the gospel by our holy conduct. We can walk worthy of the calling we have received. In this way, women, whether married or single, can be cornerstones, reflecting the glory of the chief cornerstone, Jesus Christ Himself (Eph. 2:20).

CHAPTER 17

Beauty in Your Home

As women pass through their twenties unmarried, they begin to wonder if they should establish their own home, continue to share an apartment with friends, or live with their parents. Obviously, the answer will vary, but I hope that many of these unmarried women are in a situation where they can establish a *robust Christian culture* in their own homes. Beauty has an impact on our souls and on those around us. Though a single woman may not have her own children around her table, she does not need to view herself as barren. She can make her home a warm, inviting, hospitable place. And she can have many friends and their children around her table. Unfortunately, many Christian homes (with children in them!) are barren: colorless, bleak, gloomy, and stale. Is this what we want to share with others? Is this a sample of Christian living? I have been in Christian homes where the blinds were drawn tight, where the only items in view were simply utilitarian and mostly ugly, where the sunshine was shut out, and the thermostat was turned down so low that not only was it dreary, it was cold too. All I could think was, "Get me out of here!"

Judging from the way many Christian women dress and how they set their tables, you would think our religion was one of misers, ascetics, scrooges, and grumps. There is a serious disconnect somewhere. Surely we can do better than this and get beyond decorating our homes like they were oversized cubicles.

We do not serve an austere God, but a God who delights to give us extravagance, an overflow of beauty, the abundant life (Jn. 10:10). We cannot ignore the beauty around us or think that it is irrelevant. God is teaching us all the time. It is plain ol' heresy to think that beauty is earthly and somehow less spiritual than dowdy, dumpy, and dreary. Beauty matters to God. His creation is full of it! Consider the passage in Matthew 6 where Jesus says that the lowly lilies of the field surpass even King Solomon who "in all his glory was not arrayed like one of these" (v. 29). If God bestows such beauty on His creation, surely He calls us to imitate Him in our lowly homes where we are to take dominion. We are to adorn our homes to the glory of God. A dull, drab, colorless, lifeless home does not glorify God. And this is not exclusively the domain of the married.

Let's consider a few passages of Scripture so you can see that I am not making this up. God beautifies His people, and His house is beautiful. This is certainly grounds for us to imitate Him in making our own homes (or rooms or apartments) as lovely as we are able.

God makes "everything beautiful in its time." (Eccl. 3:11)

For the LORD takes pleasure in His people; He will beautify the humble with salvation. (Ps. 149:4)

How lovely is Your tabernacle, O LORD of hosts! (Ps. 84:1)

One thing I have desired of the LORD, that will I seek: that I may dwell in the house of the LORD all the days of my life, to behold the beauty of the LORD, and to inquire in His temple. (Ps. 27:4)

And you shall make holy garments for Aaron your brother, for glory and for beauty. (Exod. 28:2)

Finally, brethren, whatever things are true . . . whatever things are lovely . . . meditate on these things. (Phil. 4:8)

A house does not equal a home. A home is full of intangibles. And if we want to build a rich, potent, Christian culture, we have to realize that our surroundings matter. We don't want to settle for mediocrity when God has given us the means to appreciate the beautiful as a way of glorifying Him. We need to start with what we have, learn to look for, to study, to appreciate the beautiful. Then we can take a look at our homes and see how to make them more beautiful. This is something that single women often overlook. Come on! You need to realize that you are a potent force in the Church, and this potency starts in your own spot, whatever that is.

Here are a few excuses I have heard.

I don't know how.

This is legitimate. Some moms have not equipped their daughters. Not knowing how is not the same as guilt. But it's time to get out there and learn. We want our children to pass us up. You may need to first pass up your own parents, your own upbringing. Ask a friend for help; read a book (like *Hidden Art* by Edith Schaeffer); take a class. Look around! Take a walk and look at older homes; they have greater aesthetic charm than modern ones. They appreciated the details of trim, wainscoting, fixtures.

I don't have time (to shop, to learn, to decorate).

This can be legitimate also. But just start small. Cut some daffodils and put them in a vase. Don't think you have to do it all at once. Start opening your eyes to the beauty around you. Learn to appreciate it first. Then you won't have the time to neglect this. You can make your bed even if you are the only one who will see it.

I don't have money.

We all have our limits. But we've all probably seen wealthy people living in sterile homes and poor people living in bright and cheery places. So even if you can't afford a leather sofa, you can clean the bathroom. Shop thrift stores and tag sales if you have to. Money isn't everything. Even so, it helps. Start a yard sale fund. Save up for new curtains, or cut up a tablecloth and sew them. Make your apartment teeming with color and life and joy. Plants are cheap and seeds are cheaper. Make some pillows. Paint works wonders.

I'm embarrassed to try.

Fear of failure is a poor excuse. Consider the many domestic arts, like knitting, sewing, gardening, cooking, flower arranging, or decorating. Just pick one, and find a friend to help you. This is not a big commitment!

Maybe your mom or grandma has some lovely dishes, linens, or furniture she would love to give you. Take it! As we recover and repair the ruins of our Christian heritage, we've had to start at the beginning, establishing right worship, figuring out how to educate our kids, taking them out of the state schools, and pretty much starting at square one. Now our children can build on that foundation, but much still needs to be done. We need women who can excel in music, painting, writing, composing, building, decorating, designing, and all the rest. God has adorned us with the gospel. Now we, by faith, can adorn our homes as an outworking of this glorious gospel.

As you do this in your own space, whatever it is, do it by faith and ask God to bless it. Ask God to give you more so that you will have more to give. He who is faithful with a little will be faithful with much.

When my daughter was unmarried, she began gathering all kinds of things for her future home. I remember her saying once, "I don't have a hope chest. I have a presumption chest!" She bought tools for her future kitchen and did not have the attitude of, "When I am married, I'll get one of those." She jumped right in at the first opportunity and began enjoying herself.

If you are not the "crafty" type, don't think I am criticizing you or saying you must be sewing your own curtains. You can cook and decorate and set a table even if you have no desire for making candles. So my word to you is this: don't wait. Jump in now and enjoy making a home. If you like to cook, then have fun in the kitchen. If you like to garden, then plant some pumpkins. The idea is to embrace your home, whatever it is, and make it a beautiful place to be.

CHAPTER 18

What About a Career?

When I was unmarried and out of college, I went to lunch with my future mother-in-law, Bessie Wilson. She had been a missionary in Japan and married Jim when she was thirty-two (he was twenty-four). During our little lunch date, I asked her whether I should be preparing to go to the mission field. I remember her wisely suggesting that I stay where I was. In fact, she told me not to rule out marriage (which continued to be our little joke). Though I had not ruled out marriage, I didn't want to just be sitting around waiting.

Many women ask me about the wisdom of pursuing a career since they don't see marriage in the immediate future. Maybe you can go to lunch with someone like Bessie to help you sort it out. Meanwhile, let me suggest a few general principles to help you think about your options.

First of all, what are your gifts, opportunities, and desires? If you have a desire to pursue nursing, and you have the opportunity, then by all means go through the door that the Lord seems to be opening for you. If you can do this without putting yourself behind the eight-ball financially, then God bless you. When it comes to medical school, which is a much bigger and more difficult commitment, I would advise more caution because of the heavy financial obligations involved, as well as the serious time commitment. If you are in your last year of med school and you meet someone you want to marry, how will you feel about leaving med school then? What about all the debt? The temptation will be to finish med school since you have already gotten this far. That might create pressure on you to sacrifice the greater good to the lesser good.

Whatever career you decide to pursue, you should be willing in principle to drop it if the right man comes along. The reason I say this is because any career that you might have is inferior to the calling you will have as a wife and mother. Remember, the biblical picture is for you to be a helper to your husband, not the other way around. If you pursue a career that does not require such a heavy investment of time and money, you may find it much easier to drop everything when a husband comes along. And sometimes, depending on your circumstances, you may not need to drop it right off the bat. So consider these things as you invest yourself in a career. When it comes to law school or med school, it may be very tough to walk away. However, if you believe you could, then go ahead, keeping an open hand before the Lord.

But consider where this will take you. Will you be in a community where you can be a member in a faithful church? You don't want to head off to the wilderness (spiritually speaking) for several years. If you want to be married, then you should want to be in a community where there is a possibility of meeting someone like-minded. My dad always told me that distance adds intrigue. But once you get there, there you are.

The other thing to think about is what kind of career it is. Is it consistent with a godly femininity? If so, that will rule out becoming a cop, a road construction worker, a race car driver, a football coach, a bouncer, or a combat officer (to mention a few). There is no reason on earth for a Christian woman to pursue such things. God has given women many gifts, talents, and abilities, so use them, and leave the men to use theirs. I realize there are many career choices that are neither masculine nor feminine, but our society wants to (and has succeeded in) blurring the edges in many that are necessarily masculine. Christian women want to think clearly about such things and grow more feminine, not less, as a result of their career choices.

CHAPTER 19

No Regrets

One of the important lessons I have learned over the years is that God seldom moves us on from one condition to another one until we have gotten the victory where we are. When my husband and I were first married, we moved into an old house that had been converted into two apartments. Though it was charming at first, it grew to be very inconvenient in many ways. And, to top it off, I developed a sour attitude toward that place. We began looking for a new place, but try as we might, nothing ever worked out. And I continued to see all the problems with our apartment.

In one of our conversations about the place, my husband wisely told me that God was not going to move us out of that place until I would be sad to leave. I was shocked! Was he kidding? But the more I thought about it, the more I realized that he was right. So I began working on my attitude and cultivating a little gratitude instead of fussing. When we did finally move out, I can't say that I shed a tear. But I did gain the victory over that place. Why should God move me out of my situation while I am fussing about it? He is trying to teach me something.

This principle has application to single women. You want to be able to look back on these years with no regrets. You don't want to be in a position of wishing you had been more joyful, more fruitful, more thankful, less stressed out, less worrisome, less dejected about your "unmarriedness." You want to move from victory to victory here and now and straight into the future. Then you'll be able to look back with gratitude and see how God's hand was in all that happened to you. He ordained it all, and He has always had a good plan for your life. Determine to live like you believe it. Then you will have no regrets.